The
WELL
WOMAN
Series

MENOPAUSE

Jan de Vries

FOREWORD BY
GLORIA HUNNIFORD

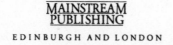
MAINSTREAM
PUBLISHING
EDINBURGH AND LONDON

First published in Great Britain in 1993 by
MAINSTREAM PUBLISHING COMPANY (EDINBURGH) LTD
7 Albany Street
Edinburgh EH1 3UG

ISBN 1 85158 448 X (cloth)
ISBN 1 85158 449 8 (paper)

A catalogue record for this book is available from the British Library

Typeset in 11/12½pt Monophoto Palatino by Servis Filmsetting Ltd, Manchester

Printed in Great Britain by BPCC Wheatons, Exeter

Contents

We move from the simple to the
  complex
The obvious is the last thing we
  learn

'A Truth'

Foreword

by *Gloria Hunniford*

EVERY SO OFTEN along comes a natural communicator and broadcaster, who immediately builds up a worthwhile relationship with the listeners and viewers. Such a man is Jan de Vries. I have worked with him on various Radio 2 and television programmes since 1984, and the mailbag or phonelines have regularly been bursting with medical queries, which he has dealt with in excellent professional terms.

However, what has clearly emerged is the number of Well Woman medical problems. Therefore, as a result of the many questions on my programmes, Jan has embarked on the Well Woman series, starting with premenstrual and menopausal conditions, to be followed with books on the subjects of childbirth and pregnancy, mother and child, skin and hair conditions, and women's cancers. These books will answer in depth the many queries that we have had on the programmes and I do hope that this series of books will be of help with many of the presently common conditions.

Gloria

Chapter 1

What is the Menopause?

THE MENOPAUSE is an important stage in the life of each woman. Some women are pleased that they have reached the end of menstruation and the unpleasant symptoms associated with it, while other women are grateful that they need no longer fear an unwanted or unplanned pregnancy. However, there are also women who believe that life after the menopause is going to be less pleasant.

The menopause is mostly associated with a period of time when women may experience diverse complaints such as hot flushes, night sweats, tiredness, anxiety, lack of energy, depression, lack of confidence, vaginal dryness, change of mood, and other less specific symptoms. However, should the menopausal period constitute a problem, much can be achieved by understanding the physiological changes that take place in the female body during this time of life, while at the same time realising that much can be done to minimise the problems.

For some women the first signs of the onset of the menopause, which occurs mostly during the mid-forties, are uncertainty and a lack of purpose about the future. The menstrual cycle becomes irregular, the production of the oestrogen hormone slowly wanes and they become aware of some of the symptoms already mentioned.

The word menopause describes the moment when a woman's fertile period approaches the end. This stage is reached when the ovaries are losing or have lost the ability to perform the major part of their function, i.e. the production of ova (eggs) and the oestrogen hormone. The menopause therefore signifies the end of an extremely important stage in the life of women. However, never doubt that the post-menopausal period holds much in store and should be regarded as a new phase in your life.

Let me remind you of the fact that in earlier centuries the life expectancy was such that women rarely reached the age of 40 and therefore hardly anything was known about the menopause. At the beginning of the nineteenth century the expected lifespan for women was 48 years. Since then better health care and diet have combined to create a much longer life expectancy. Statistics show that at present in the Western world the average age reached by a woman is around 78, and, bearing in mind that the menopause occurs in one's late forties or early fifties, this indicates that a third of a woman's life is still ahead of her after the menopause.

How the menopausal period is experienced by individual women depends a great deal on the measure of balance achieved during the years of menstruation. Are you a stressful person by nature? Do you receive support from your husband, family and friends? Are you comfortable discussing your problems with your doctor? Contrary to popular belief most women pass through the menopause without any significant problems, although fully aware of the physiological changes. Other women require general or expert help and guidance in order to be able to accept and cope with the changes that take place in the body during this stage. Hot flushes and night sweats can result in lack of sleep and general tiredness, making a woman irritable and nervous. She is therefore less capable of concentrating and as a result lacks decisiveness. It is an unfortunate fact that men often also pass through a period of increased uncertainty at this stage of their lives, and therefore neither partner may be able to offer the level of support that is sought and expected.

At this stage it is often decided to seek medical advice and

10

frequently a supplementary oestrogen preparation is prescribed. I wonder if this is always necessary. Although HRT (Hormone Replacement Therapy) has benefits, I fear that the body is often not given the time to find a new balance in the way nature would, if given the chance. Nature will run its own course and will readily establish its own levels for compensation of physiological shortages and changes. It is often not recognised that naturopathy offers an alternative and less aggressive approach. It may require no more than a change in dietary habits to counteract a calcium deficiency or lack of vitamin absorption, all of which can be easily overcome.

A lack of confidence at this stage in a woman's life is often caused because they feel they are losing their appeal to the opposite sex and if nothing else a substitute hormone supplement may at least slow down the development of wrinkles and delay the possible onset of osteoporosis. However, it has not been proved beyond any doubt that these preparations are free of side-effects. If it is at all possible, why shouldn't we give nature a chance first? Having said this, I must immediately refute the idea that women of this age are less attractive to men. It is widely recognised that they often exert a greater appeal because of their maturity and wisdom. It is a great pity that the term menopause or change of life is so often misinterpreted. Admittedly it is the end of a woman's reproductive years, but during the next stage of life women have so many other gifts to offer. Psychologically, the more positive a woman is about the change of life, the better she will cope with this period. How well she copes largely depends on her own approach and the understanding of her husband and her immediate family. If a husband or family's understanding is lacking or withheld, emotional and erratic moodiness may occur and it is not unusual that during this stage of her life a woman may feel emotionally deserted and therefore experience greater physical menopause problems than would have been the case if she had received solid support.

For all concerned it is important to understand the primary hormonal functions. The production of hormones is all important in the reproductive process, but they are also active in other bodily functions. Hormones are substances that are produced by the body and have the role of messengers. The word 'hormone' is derived from Greek and means 'to excite'. Every form of life produces hormones –

humans, animals and plants alike – although biologically the hormonal messengers produce different results, depending upon the species. Each hormone stimulates organs, tissue or body functions in its own specific way.

Of the better known hormones, the oestrogen hormone belongs to a group of several female sex hormones, while testosterone is a male sex hormone, and progesterone is a steroid hormone that prepares the uterus for the fertilised ovum and the mammary glands for milk secretion. The ovaries produce both oestrogen and progesterone, which in differing quantities are deposited in the bloodstream during the monthly cycle. The ovaries also produce a small quantity of testosterone. On average once every four weeks an egg (or ovum) is released after ovulation and by way of the oviduct or Fallopian tube this egg reaches the womb. When sperm enters the womb via the cervix impregnation may take place. The womb is an organ with a length of about 8cm where the fertilised egg can develop into a foetus. The lining of the womb, where the fertilised egg will settle, is called the endometrium. However, when the egg has not been fertilised, it will be disposed of during the monthly menstruation when the lining of the womb is discarded.

There are two organs that are capable of hormone production which are utilised in the reproductive system.

The first is the pituitary gland, at the base of the brain, which produces two hormones that are influential in the procreative cycle. These are referred to as FSH and LH (follicle stimulating hormone and luteinising hormone). The adrenals, one of which is found just above each of the kidneys, produce hormones during one's entire life, which are converted into oestrogen and testosterone. This source of oestrogen is especially important during the post-menopausal period, because the ovaries are no longer capable of producing oestrogen.

Second is the hypothalamus, a gland placed just above the pituitary gland, which acts as the control centre for the production of FSH and LH by way of the pituitary.

On average a woman's fertility begins to wane in her early forties when ovulation may start to become slightly irregular. During this stage unplanned pregnancies are not unheard of because ovulation still takes place, although in an irregular pattern. Remember that at this point one is ill-advised to practise the natural rhythm method, because the regularity of ovulation may have disappeared and it would therefore be wise to take extra care in contraceptive methods. The actual production of oestrogen during the years of the menopause differs considerably among individuals. When ovulation stops progesterone is no longer produced, which results in reduced oestrogen production. This can lead to a thickening of the lining of the womb, slightly increasing the risk of cancer. When unusual blood loss is experienced the doctor is therefore likely to advise a minor surgical performance commonly called 'D and C' (dilatation and curettage), or a course of supplementary progesterone.

The monthly menstruation cycle may well have stopped, yet, due to the continual production of oestrogen, the symptoms one has come to associate with the monthly cycle may still be experienced, e.g. swelling of the breasts and a tendency to retain fluids. These symptoms can be controlled by dietary changes, diuretics or indeed by a low progesterone supplement in order to slow down oestrogen production. Then a new cycle begins which shows itself as a blood loss that resembles menstruation. It is also possible that the doctor would advise a combination of oestrogen and progesterone in order to control the blood loss.

When ovulation no longer takes place and menstruation stops, the following menopausal symptoms are frequently experienced:

Hot flushes: One of the most frequently experienced symptoms of the menopause, probably caused by a reduced production of oestrogen. This influences the autonomic nervous system that dictates the functioning of the capillaries in the skin. Due to occasional increases in the blood supply, blushing is experienced, often combined with sudden hot flushes and sweats. These can vary from once or twice a month to 15 or 20 times a day. Although uncomfortable for the person who is subjected to hot flushes, they are nevertheless harmless. Make sure that you wear comfortable and loose clothes, preferably cotton, because this allows the heat to escape easily.

Night sweats: Another manifestation of the changes leading to hot flushes during the day. The heat and moisture is contained under the bedclothes causing one to wake up clammy or cold. Like the hot flushes, the night sweats are harmless, although the unfortunate result is a disturbed night, which can easily be the cause of tiredness and irritability.

Heart palpitations: This is often described as a frightening experience, but is primarily caused by a sudden increase in the blood supply.

Pains, weakness and stiffness: Emotional tension and stress can cause muscular cramping in the back and neck. Stiffness is caused by a lack of physical exercise, which can cause fluid retention in the legs. These complaints can be easily overcome by exercise and relaxation.

Weight increase: After the menopause women only require two-thirds of their previous calorie intake. Food is utilised more slowly by the body and fat deposits seem to settle, specifically around the stomach, hips, back and shoulders. By eating less fatty food and salt, excessive weight increase can be avoided during this time.

Wrinkles: The skin structure changes as a result of the reduced oestrogen production. If you lose weight after the menopause extra wrinkles will appear. Too much sunshine on an unprotected skin can also cause dryness and encourage the formation of wrinkles. However, let's not forget that wrinkles are an inevitable part of the ageing process.

Flatulence and irregular bowel movements: A further effect of the reduced oestrogen production is a slowing down in the function of the intestines, possibly causing flatulence and less regular bowel movements. Adapt your diet to compensate for this, but if the problems persist consult your doctor.

Concentration problems: In general the memory lapses women complain about during the menopause arise because women tend to worry more during this time, are more easily distracted and less able to concentrate.

Depressions: It is not unusual for a woman to feel depressed, especially if she lacks the understanding or support of her husband and family. A little extra care or attention from someone dear to you will mostly lighten the depression.

A basic homoeopathic principle is that man has three different aspects: physical, mental and emotional. The health of any of these aspects is dependent on the health of the other two. In this context it is important that the menopausal problem is approached in a holistic way as each of these aspects is closely linked to the hormone system by way of the endocrine system, which can only be treated through the emotional aspect. In holistic medicine the aim is to attain harmony within these three aspects. The emotional aspect is probably the most important here, because the physiological and emotional changes of the menopause period may be numerous. It would be unwise to confuse some of the effects of the menopause with aspects of mental illness, even though stress due to physiological and emotional changes becomes more noticeable and exaggerated. The menopause is a completely normal and natural occurrence and must not be turned into some sort of disease. It should be viewed as the beginning of a new stage of life, on a par with puberty, or motherhood. This stage of life, like the others, offers new opportunities and a measure of freedom not previously experienced.

Remember, I am not saying that one should ignore or misinterpret the physical messages emitted by the body. In some of my books, e.g. *Body Energy*, or *Cancer and Leukaemia*, I have mentioned external signs where the body tries to draw our attention to something. Although a positive outlook is always essential, there are certain messages which you simply must not ignore. In this category I would again mention heavy and prolonged blood loss, because this may be overcome easily by a minor surgical operation and much discomfort may be avoided. If this is brought to the doctor's attention and timely action is taken, it may severely reduce the risk of cancer of the womb or the cervix (the neck of the womb). I would also strongly advise self-examination of the breasts and please take advantage of the opportunity for regular smear tests. Much recrimination may be avoided by an awareness of these facts and a sensible and responsible attitude to one's own health.

The post-menopausal period is not necessarily like a second youth. During the menopause the body becomes accustomed to a reduced oestrogen concentration, but some of the effects of this may not become apparent until after the menopause. One example of this is that the previously regular oestrogen production ensured that the vaginal wall remained strong and elastic, producing sufficient vaginal fluids. However, due to the reduced oestrogen supply, changes will take place in the vagina. This will gradually become narrower and less elastic, and also produce less moisture. In medical terms this is referred to as 'vaginal atrophy'. Depending upon the oestrogen concentration, these effects will become more noticeable over a number of years following the menopause. This can be the cause of some embarrassment, discomfort or pain during sexual intercourse, and also increase the risk of vaginal infections. Do not suffer, but ask your doctor or practitioner for advice.

Another problem frequently experienced is reduced bladder control. Again, as a result of the reduced oestrogen concentration the muscles and connective tissue in the pelvic area grow less elastic. A weak bladder is more prone to infection and because of muscle weakness in the intestinal area bowel movements may be less frequent. The walls of the urethra become weaker and this is the reason why women could experience slight incontinence problems when laughing, sneezing or coughing. Consult your doctor if you experience frequent urges to pass water or cannot control your bladder, because this may point to a form of urinary infection. Because of general weakening of the muscles the womb may have dropped to an uncomfortable position where it is pressing on the bladder and, if this is the case, your doctor may advise the use of a vaginal pessary to relieve the pressure or it may be suggested that you undergo a surgical operation, depending on the severity of the situation.

Starting in the early forties the bone density of women begins to wane. From the menopause onwards this process speeds up and the bones become more brittle and the risk of broken bones increases. This occurrence is known as osteoporosis. Approximately half of all women become subject to a higher risk of osteoporosis during the post-menopausal period. However, let it be said that women who are physically active are less prone to this disease than those who take insufficient physical exercise. The first signs of osteoporosis may not become apparent during the first ten years or so after the menopause. Initially the pain is likely to start in the back and when the osteoporosis becomes more advanced, even a relatively minor injury can result in a fractured bone. Nowadays this condition, when recognised, even with a family history, is mostly treated with supplementary oestrogen in combination with progesterone. However, to avoid osteoporosis it is very important to take exercise. This need not be strenuous, but gentle exercise is recommended such as walking, swimming or cycling, which can be continued to an advanced age. Dietary measures include calcium-rich foods, or a calcium supplement. Vitamin D is also important and it is good to remember that fish, butter, eggs and liver are good sources.

As a result of reduced concentration of oestrogen, women may discover a change in their hair. Usually the quality deteriorates slightly and it is not uncommon for a hair growth on the upper lip or chin to become noticeable. This growth is due to the presence of the male hormone testosterone in the body. After the menopause oestrogen concentration in the body is insufficient to counter the function of testosterone. Do not worry unduly because these unwanted hairs can be removed or bleached and if necessary this effect can be undone by a small oestrogen supplement.

During the menopause some women develop an under-active thyroid. Why this should be so is not known, but this appears to be more prevalent in the later years. The classic symptoms are constipation, slowness of speech, hoarseness, intolerance to cold, puffiness, thickening or scaling of the skin and reflex problems. Early detection can forestall many problems, thereby preventing more major problems.

Having discussed some of the possible side-effects of the menopause, let me reassure you that many women suffer none or very few of these symptoms while going through this stage in their lives. The first rule is that this phase is seen in a positive light and that it should be viewed as the beginning of a new stage, rather than the end of an earlier stage. The value of positive thinking is reflected in the words of the well-known author, R. D. Grandville: 'If you don't want trouble, don't think it and don't say it. Words are thoughts with a birth certificate. Once said, they are firmly recorded.'

An understanding of the menopause and some knowledge of the physiology of the ovarian system will help to allay our fears. Nature never ceases to amaze me. Consider that at birth a baby girl already has two ovaries, containing about 150,000 microscopic egg cells. Most of these eggs die off during childhood and at the onset of puberty the ovaries, which have grown to approximately the size of an almond, contain about 25,000 eggs. Only very few of these many eggs are ever fertilised and it is astounding that nature has provided the body with this large number of eggs. Only one egg needs to be fertilised by male sperm to produce a child. It is a miracle that since birth a baby girl is equipped with these internal organs and from puberty onwards has the ability to create new life and happiness.

Although hormone supplements have their use, it must be remembered that there are disadvantages as well as advantages. It has been claimed that oestrogen supplements could possibly be the cause of an increased risk of cancer of the breast, womb or cervix, of gall-bladder problems, thrombosis, diabetes or high blood pressure. The statistics on which these conclusions were based stem from the early years of hormone supplements. Even so, women who have previously been treated for breast cancer or cancer of the womb should not be considered as candidates for hormone supplements.

It is also important to keep an eye on the cardio-vascular system as women in their fifties are more prone to develop cardio-vascular problems. This could lead to increased risk of a stroke and hypertension. The risk factor at this particular age can be curtailed by not smoking or drinking, sensible physical exercise and weight and cholesterol checks. Menopausal anxiety, irritability and insomnia need to be recognised for what they are at this stage and then steps can be taken to overcome these problems. Over the years I have prescribed a variety of herbal remedies and some of the menopause formulae of Dr Vogel like MNP, or the Woman's Formula, can be of tremendous help. For insomnia Dormeasan – 40 drops last thing at night – will be of great help. Menopausal fatigue and depression can be helped with herbal remedies and Zincum valerianicum D3 is often of tremendous help. The gentle action of herbs will help to soothe and relieve irritations, infections or anxieties. Mineral supplements, dietary changes and natural enzymes may bring welcome relief and they are often an effective means of balancing and optimising one's nutritional intake.

Chapter 2

Menstrual Bleeding and Irregular Periods

IN THE PERIOD leading up to the menopause, the menstrual flow may fluctuate, temporarily increasing or decreasing, although sometimes there is little or no change from the usual pattern. Variations may range from scanty or short to long or heavy menstrual periods. If the changes are drastic and unsettling it is wise to seek medical advice. I have had patients who claimed that the flow sometimes was so heavy that it was almost impossible to stay dry for even a minute. If the bleeding is very heavy it is essential to seek a doctor's or gynaecologist's advice, because if the situation is allowed to get out of control it will sap the energy very quickly. The bleeding may periodically change from heavy to light, but do not allow this to continue without a medical check. Prolonged bleeding spells can lead to anaemia, which is a decrease of haemoglobin and the iron-containing molecules in the blood which carry oxygen. Anaemia can lead to listlessness, lethargy and weakness, usually accompanied by a pale and colourless complexion.

Another problem is when bleeding occurs between periods, or

bleeding in women who no longer menstruate. This could be a sign of cancer of the reproductive organs and therefore should never be neglected.

During the menopause women often experience change in the menstrual cycle. Although some women stop menstruating very suddenly, these changes more often than not take place over months or even years. If medical advice is required it is always helpful to provide the specialist with a definite picture of the change in pattern of the menstrual cycle. Therefore it is sometimes considered helpful to keep a record of the menstrual pattern prior to and during the menopause. Too often I have heard women tell me that they lived in constant dread of pregnancy during the menopause. They frequently take pregnancy tests and as the cyclical pattern becomes more and more unreliable, they should consider reliable contraceptive methods. Pregnancy tests are often taken because some symptoms of the menopause may resemble those experienced in early pregnancy, such as breast tenderness, nausea, fatigue, etc.

Flooding or heavy bleeding can disrupt one's life to such an extent that a woman feels she lacks control though, in the case of heavy bleeding, something can be done. It does not make sense to put up with it for a few months, because soon it will all be over. The body instinctively signals when something is not as it should be and it is absolutely wrong to ignore these signs. When these signals occur it is quite possible that much suffering can be avoided if the problems are treated at an early stage. There is sometimes insecurity during this period of life and a change in the menstrual pattern raises many questions in a woman's mind, the most common of which are:

'Is it normal at my age that my periods are so close together and so heavy?'
'I hardly dare leave the house because I never know when I will next start flooding.'
'Some time ago my periods suddenly stopped, but I know that this cannot be the end of it and I am scared that I will suddenly be caught out.'
'Although I no longer menstruate I have these dreadful night sweats.'

Each woman experiences the menopause in her own way, which does not mean that the experiences of others cannot be of help. The body produces hormones – oestrogen and progesterone – according to a pattern, but because of the so-called 'change of life', there is an imbalance. Ovulation takes place with less regularity and the hormonal output varies. Towards the age of fifty, menstrual periods are likely to come with increasing irregularity, after which they will stop entirely. Although the menopause can cause some problems one should regard this phase positively. Appreciate that after so many years the menstrual cycle is over and enjoy a new-found freedom. From a positive viewpoint it is a phase when many habitual sufferers of headaches or migraines may outgrow them. It is no longer necessary to dread pelvic discomfort, pregnancy, PMS, fibroid tumours, or to practise birth control. However, if you have a real concern about the menstrual changes that are taking place, seek medical advice. Continuous heavy blood loss should be treated as it could prevent the necessity of a dilatation and curettage at a later stage. A D and C is a minor surgical operation that will stop the bleeding, and medical attention at that time may indicate possible causes for the bleeding, sometimes even recognised as the early stages of cancer of the reproductive organs or the abdomen.

The D and C procedure involves the removal of the lining of the uterus, usually by suction or scraping, while the patient is either under local or general anaesthetic. The cells are analysed for any abnormal patterns, but if a menstrual problem is due to a hormonal imbalance leading up to the menopause, the same symptoms may recur. In that case excessive bleeding will often be treated with a progesterone hormone supplement.

At this point I would like to add that such problems can also be overcome by natural means and, under guidance, this is often the preferred method. Few people ever think of studying the characteristics of plants, herbs, flowers, roots or leaves. If we did this more often we would soon realise the value of some of the treasure supplied by nature. Often the characteristics of plants and herbs are a subtle means of identifying for which specific purpose they may be used. A good example for heavy blood loss is the *Hamamelis virginiana* and for many centuries this has been used for heavy bleeding. In the eighteenth and nineteenth centuries the Indians brought these medicinal virtues to the notice of European settlers, although it was not until 1882 that this wonderful plant was first mentioned in the United States *Pharmacopoeia* for just this purpose. This plant beckons with its young flowery twigs which contain clear astringent properties for heavy blood flow. According to medical folklore *Hamamelis virginiana* is useful for the treatment of haemorrhages of the rectum, the nose and the uterus, and also externally for haemorrhoids and varicose veins. As an astringent it is also an efficient means of controlling heavy menstrual bleeding. Nature's subtle messages should not be ignored. The common name of *Hamamelis virginiana* is witch hazel and this plant contains wonderful medicinal properties.

This is not all the herbal kingdom has to offer. Tormentavena is a mixture of herbs containing tormentil, loosestrife, hemp nettle, knotweed, oats and butterbur and is like a bouquet of herbs, not only capable of preventing abnormal menstrual bleeding, but also for the treatment of bleeding haemorrhoids and inflammation of the mucous membranes. Tormentavena is also recommended for internal bleeding which may occur as a result of painful sexual intercourse. Heavy and prolonged menstrual bleeding can cause anaemia and the effect of this can be counteracted by natural remedies, such as Alfavena which contains alfalfa extract, stinging nettle and oat seed extract. This combination is very effective for preventing iron deficiency. If iron deficiency is diagnosed a stronger remedy with a higher iron content is necessary. Iron is one of the most common nutritional deficiencies among women, because the iron contained in the blood cells, which is otherwise recycled, is lost during menstruation. Iron is essential for all life processes, as without it oxygen cannot be transported around the body. It is also a component of enzymes and is needed for the metabolism of the B vitamins. In some cases I advise Nature's Best Vital B-Complex. This supplement contains essential nutrients which take part in iron assimilation and encourages more efficient absorption. Encapsulated with gelatin, glycerin and water, each capsule provides:

Vitamin C	100mg
Vitamin B	10mg
Vitamin B_2	10mg

Nicotinamide	60mg
Vitamin B_6 hydrochloride	10mg
Vitamin B_{12}	10mcg
Pantothenic acid	80mg
Folic acid	400mcg
Biotin	100mcg
Choline	150mg
PABA	20mg
Inositol	150mg
Pangamic acid	30mg

The same manufacturer also produces a supplement of Natural Iron with Blackstrap Molasses. One good thing to come out of refining sugar is the trace nutrient-rich syrup that is left behind. This is called molasses and it is an ideal ingredient for an iron gluconate remedy. Each tablet of Natural Iron with Blackstrap Molasses contains 25mg chelated iron in a base of blackstrap molasses. This remedy is a worthwhile supplement for women who, because of heavy menstrual bleeding, risk becoming anaemic.

Quite often I feel that at this stage in a woman's life extra zinc is necessary. Soil deficiencies of zinc have reduced the levels available in plant foods, and zinc is also removed by food processing. High levels of calcium and phytates found in plant foods are thought to block absorption of zinc from food. The body's stores of zinc may be threatened by missing meals or fasting. The most reliable sources of zinc are shellfish, herrings and meat, and many vegetarians and people who eat a wholefood diet choose to supplement with zinc. Smokers, alcohol drinkers, users of the contraceptive pill, the elderly and athletes (zinc is lost in perspiration) may also take extra zinc.

Zinc is well known for its role in growth and tissue repair and essential for the immune system. It is vital that children and adolescents receive enough zinc. Not only is it required for overall growth, but especially for the healthy function of reproductive organs.

Even more importantly, zinc is involved in hundreds of metabolic pathways. Some of these pathways maintain vision and our senses of smell and taste. Others deal with the digestion of carbohydrates and the balance of insulin which controls the blood-sugar, the absorption of other nutrients, such as vitamin A and the B-complex vitamins, and cell metabolism. As part of many different chemical catalysts, or enzymes, zinc is one of our most important antioxidants, as part of the major antioxidant enzyme super-oxide dismutase (SOD), and it protects cells from the damage caused by oxidising fats.

Having treated many patients, I am very aware of the possible energy-draining effects of heavy menstrual bleeding and irregular periods and I have worked out a few important laws especially designed for women at the menopausal stage. Always try to take some exercise in the fresh air, so as to receive plenty of oxygen. As stated, this is not only an essential part of life, it also attracts iron to the body. For the sake of your health, bear in mind the following Five Laws of Life:

Oxidisation is the keystone of health. Life is in the blood. Oxygen is the bridge between life and death, between health and disease.

Elimination is the removal of waste. The accumulation of waste in the body with its toxic by-products would kill anyone in 24 hours.

Nutrition. The building and repair of the body. The energy to function is maintained by the use of oxygen in the tissues.

Motion or Vibration. Expansion and contraction of cells, muscles and tissues.

Relaxation. The least expenditure of energy, while keeping the body functioning.

Remember that the blood is purified by oxygen in the lungs. People in poor health always lack oxygen in their blood. No bacteria can live in pure oxygen or pure blood. If the respiratory tract is obstructed in any way, oxygen starvation results, leading not only to disease in the open cavities in the nose, throat and ears, but also in the closed cavities elsewhere in the body.

Five most important functions of oxygen

1. It has combustible units of gas that give off heat. These units of heat make soluble nutritional elements fit for absorption in the body.
2. Vapour or water that keeps the gas in solution has a dissolving power greater than any other element entering the body. This

moisture, combined with heat, melts secretions and renders them liquid for elimination.

3. Oxygen attracts iron to the body. This is one of the essential elements for stamina and virility.
4. Oxygen maintains cell rate activity.
5. Oxygen is needed by the sinuses and contributes to balance and resonance of the voice.

Almost all bacterial diseases are due to lack of oxygen and the function of oxygen in the open cavities of the head or in the closed cavities of the body is necessary to health. *Oxidation is Life*. You can be paralysed and live, but you cannot live without oxygen, no matter how many adjustments you make. The rate of exchange may be fast or slow, but the process of exchange of carbon dioxide for oxygen is continuous, ending only at death.

The life of a woman can have some very interesting milestones: first love, engagement, marriage, birth of the children, the children's puberty, the menopause, and after the menopause life can become very much easier. Very often financial worries are less, the understanding between husband and wife improves and it can be an exciting episode in a woman's life if a few things are taken into account. Women often seem frightened that the menopause will cause them to lose their figure. They fear that their hair may change, they will turn grey, and that they will become less attractive. This is a distressingly pessimistic outlook as many problems can be forestalled or overcome by taking some preventative or remedial steps. This brings me to the subject of irregular periods.

The beginning of the menopause is often signalled by irregular menstrual periods and when this phase is reached, there is no need to despair because there are ways to deal with this. Earlier I explained that the body consists of three fields of energy. In effect we have three bodies: the physical, mental and the emotional body. Emotions at this particular time of life can have a profound effect on the reproductive system.

You may wonder why there is so much more talk about the menopause than there used to be. Could it be that a more comfortable lifestyle has made us less hardy? It is nothing like that, because the reasons are much more obvious. In times past health problems, and especially women's health problems, would never be the topic of an open discussion. Moreover, it used to be quite normal for women to produce children well into their forties and generally they died at a much earlier age than is the case nowadays. Often premature death was caused by childbirth. The average life expectancy has greatly increased in recent years. But stresses, strains and financial worries affect the whole system and all three bodies are very much involved in a change of life. Although all mechanisms are at work, the negativity, which is so easily experienced during this phase of a woman's life, will prolong negative emotions. The area of the brain that controls ovarian function may not operate in the same way; ovulation becomes irregular and almost certainly there will be a hormonal imbalance.

Sometimes it is difficult to find an easy answer, but there are benefits in giving the body what, to all intents and purposes, amounts to a bit of shock treatment. If this is done positively, one can acquire greatly improved health. Why shouldn't a smoker give up smoking, or a drinker give up alcohol? These are good resolutions and positive action will provide a positive result. Nobody is helped by excessive reliance upon coffee, tea, chocolate or Coca-Cola. One lady who sought my help told me that she drank between six to eight pints of Coca-Cola every day. The caffeine content of this addictive liquid probably acted as a stimulant and the effects on her were noticeable in her weight, as well as her general outlook on life. Many a personality has been changed because of what is often thought to be an innocent indulgence or a 'quick fix'. I wonder if anyone ever gives a second thought to what caffeine does to the reproductive system. Nowadays many doctors believe that during this mid-life crisis tension or hypersensitivity may increase and many women have found that a reduction in the excessive use of these particular products will make it easier to cope with the physiological changes that take place during the menopause. It is nonsense to believe that such addictions help to calm the nerves. More often it is a question of temporarily releasing some extra stress or tension which can be achieved much more easily without dependency on stimulants.

Oddly enough, it is at this stage that many women start thinking of using the contraceptive pill, even though they may never before have felt the need. They seem to think that this may help them to cope better with some of these temporary problems. They conveniently forget that severe metabolic disturbances can actually be caused by the use of the contraceptive pill, and I would seriously advise against it, as it often causes more problems than it solves. Often the opposite happens, and physical and emotional problems, especially in the early months of using the contraceptive pill, can aggravate the symptoms. This could result in a shift of fluids retained by the body or a complete change in eating habits. The adrenals become exhausted by an over-active sympathetic nervous system or poor nutrition, and liver or kidney problems may occur. When this happens something else must be done to regain a balance. The same applies to hormone replacement therapy, which is often taken to prevent certain symptoms.

We should bear in mind that healthy women are less likely to experience menopausal problems. It is vitally important that during this period of life women should try to keep as healthy as possible, and in order to do so, the diet deserves extra consideration, so that the body can cope with the ongoing changes. In my book *Nature's Gift of Food*, the reader will find general dietary information as well as several specific diets for particular purposes.

Irregular menstrual bleeding can lead to the development of fibroids. Many women of a certain age group have been affected by fibroid cysts or uterine fibroids and although these are mostly non-malignant, their growth is stimulated by ovarian hormones, especially oestrogen. Such fibroids may cause pressure on the bowel or bladder and heavy menstrual bleeding or irregular bleeding may necessitate treatment for these fibroids. It is at this time that the remedy Petasan is beneficial. This remedy contains *Viscum album* (mistletoe) and *Petasites officinalis* (butterbur) and should be used together with large quantities of vitamin C and the remedy Urticalcin. The latter is a priceless homoeopathic calcium and silicic acid combination. The use of these remedies will often prevent the need for surgical procedures for the removal of fibroids or cysts. Essential fatty acids (which I will discuss in more detail in a later chapter) are required at all times. Sources include Oil of Evening Primrose, borage oil, blackcurrant seed oil and cod liver oil. Fibroids can grow unexpectedly large and undoubtedly are often the cause of irregular menstrual bleeding. In such instances acupuncture can be helpful, but there is a relatively new treatment method which is most effective:

the beam of a surgical laser is used to destroy the uterine lining, mostly removing the fibroids permanently. Since fibroids often develop in the stages immediately prior to the menopause or in its early stages, the fear of no longer being able to produce children is hardly relevant. Most gynaecologists are capable of performing this minor surgical operation which is occasionally done for out-patients, or incurring only a brief overnight stay in hospital. As a naturopath I like to give nature a chance first and try to overcome such problems in the natural way. However, as there are no side-effects with the laser treatment, understandably this method is often preferred because of its immediate efficacy.

At all times prevention is better than cure and problems that may indicate carcinogenic tendencies of the uterus lining or of the cervix become apparent mostly in unusually heavy or irregular menstrual periods and should therefore never be ignored.

As a protective method, women are well advised to use the Nature's Best remedy Gynovite Plus which has been designed for a woman's specific needs. For women over 40 the standard multi-vitamin and mineral formulae are often inadequate: Gynovite Plus is a unique multi-supplement whose special combination of vitamins helps to provide fine tuning. Each tablet contains:

Vitamin A	250mcg (833iu)
Thiamin (vitamin B_1)	1.7mg
Riboflavin (vitamin B_2)	1.7mg
Vitamin B_6 (pyridoxine)	3.3mg
Vitamin B_{12}	21mcg
Biotin	21mcg
Folic acid	66.7mcg
Inositol	4.2mg
Niacin (as in niacinamide)	3.3mg
Pantothenic acid	1.7mg
Para-aminobenzoic acid	4.2mg
Vitamin C	30mg
Rutin	4.2mg
Hesperidin	5.8mg
Vitamin D (as D_3)	66.7iu
Vitamin E	66.7iu

Pancreatin	15.7mg
Boron	500mcg
Calcium	83.3mg
Betaine hydrochloride	16.7mg
Chromium	33.3mcg
Copper	33.3mcg
Iodine	3mg
Magnesium	100mg
Manganese	1.7mg
Selenium	33.3mcg
Zinc	2.5mg

In a properly balanced diet vitamins and minerals are a major requirement for good health. Unfortunately, there is a tendency for modern foods to contain fewer and fewer vitamins. Growers know they can produce healthy-looking lettuce if they add cheap lime and nitrate to the soil, even though it does not contain any zinc or manganese. Supermarkets know that they need not ask too many questions, since most people will buy vegetables if they look right. Modern food processing and storage practices reduce the nutrient content of fresh, whole foods. For most of us, food gathering and preparation doesn't take even second place in the list of demands on our time: work, family, and finances come first. Even good quality, nutrient-rich food must be carefully prepared and not over-cooked if it is to retain its vitamin and mineral goodness. In addition, our way of life or physiological condition may mean we need extra nutrients. British women have turned to Optivite in increasing numbers following trials arranged by the Women's Nutritional Advisory Service, which have emphasised that Optivite works best as part of a complete health-building programme that includes adequate exercise, proper diet and effective rest and relaxation.

These are just a few hints on how to cope with problems associated with menstrual bleeding and get through the menopause as painlessly as possible. I have treated many women over the years who have been grateful for the natural remedies to ease their transition from one phase in their lives to the next.

Chapter 3

Hot Flushes

NOT SO VERY long ago, I took part in a lecture tour in the United States. One glorious morning, before my next meeting, I took a walk along the white sand of a beautiful beach in Clearwater, Florida. I watched the big waves of the Gulf of Mexico coming in and the sun was shining brightly. I felt totally relaxed, at ease and in tune with nature. While I stood there drinking in the majestic scenery, a lady of about my age walked towards me. She was dressed in a bikini and visibly enjoyed the sunshine that had tanned her skin beautifully and she must have wondered what a strange person was doing on the beach, dressed formally in a sober suit. I had only gone there to breathe in some fresh air and to enjoy the beauty of my surroundings. Although I travel all over the world, my main regret is that I rarely have any time to myself to do any sightseeing. Mostly the time I spend in these faraway places is over-subscribed.

The lady then started a conversation and asked me if I was not going to sunbathe and I told her that I had to leave in a few minutes to give a lecture. In my life there is little time for sunbathing. She then immediately wanted to know what I did for a living and when I told her, her face clouded over and she begged me for advice. She wanted to know how to cope with the awful hot flushes that plagued her day and night. In fact, she told me, they seemed to be even worse on the beach. She so much wanted to enjoy her holiday, but all day long, at regular intervals, she had to go for dips in the ocean to cool off. In her situation the worst problem of the menopause was the hot flushes.

My hotel was right on the beach and I had walked up to the beach through hotel grounds where I had seen something of interest. In the border I had found some beautiful herbs and plants and I told this lady that nature has an answer for everything. As it was nearby I invited her to walk back to the hotel with me so that I could explain something to her. She looked me up and down briefly and must have decided that I was harmless, because she accompanied me. In the hotel grounds, in one of the herbaceous borders, I showed her a plant which is primarily known as a culinary herb. Yet it is also one of the finest remedies for hot flushes. I wanted to show her the herb's healing properties and, at the same time, to demonstrate that nature gives us clues, if only we interpret the signals correctly. So I pointed to the leaves. Now that the sun had grown hot, they were perspiring just as heavily as the lady. Just as women get hot and bothered during the menopause, so this plant gets hot and bothered in the full sun and little specks of perspiration almost shout out the message that it's nature's gift to enable us to counteract hot flushes. That very special herb is known as sage or *Salvia officinalis*. This herb is known to combat any form of inflammation and also excessive perspiration, but unfortunately it is rarely considered as a treatment for night sweats. Yet it does such a wonderful job. Once during a radio programme with Gloria Hunniford I mentioned the suitability of this herb for just that purpose and I received many letters during the following months, telling me how much help this wonderful remedy had been.

What actually causes these hot flushes? Their sudden occurrence is an outward sign of a natural process women pass through in their late forties. The end of menstrual periods and increased sensitivity to extremes of heat and cold can cause the entire body to become hot and flushed. This experience can last for quite some time and, especially during the night, these flushes can be quite extreme. It is not unusual to hear a woman claim that she feels bathed in sweat. It is rarely possible to counteract this feeling with a dip in the sea, like the lady I met at Clearwater Beach. Most women consider themselves lucky if they have the opportunity of a cool shower. Fortunately these awkward symptoms do not persist for too long. Women are often embarrassed if it happens in company, as it is a visible sign of getting older. Sometimes women live in dread of hot flushes, in which case they may be inviting trouble, as the body sometimes reacts to one's thoughts.

When the output of natural oestrogen, produced by the ovaries, begins to decrease, it is to be hoped that this decrease of oestrogen is gradual, in which case the symptoms are likely to be less severe. However, if a woman is subject to hot flushes, this ought to be considered in the diet. Avoid hotly spiced meals, alcohol, nicotine and excessive heat. It doesn't make sense to do what the lady on the beach did. Instead of taking it easy in the air-conditioned hotel room, she insisted on getting a suntan. It would have been more sensible to choose cooler surroundings. It is also important to try and avoid stressful and emotional influences and to keep the brain occupied with something worthwhile. A certain area in the brain regulates the body temperature, keeping it within the range of 36–37 degrees Celsius and this thermostat in the brain is dependant upon the hormonal balance in the pituitary gland and the ovaries. Diet is important and certain forms of medication and the contraceptive pill can be decisive factors in the frequency and intensity of the hot flushes.

Urticalcin and Oil of Evening Primrose should be taken for long-term benefit, while for immediate effect it is advisable to take Salvia. Generally the calcium level of women in the menopause tends to be low. Although there are many calcium preparations, I can think of very few which I categorically believe are well absorbed into the bloodstream. It is sometimes doubtful whether the selected calcium supplement is given the chance to enter the blood stream and start its allotted task. The pioneer of traditional medicine, Dr Alfred Vogel, had his doubts, and explored the situation relentlessly before he created his calcium preparation Urticalcin. One day, deep in thought, he sat staring out of the window and suddenly realised that he was looking at a bunch of stinging nettles. He immediately knew that he had found the solution: he knew that if he were to fall into that patch of stinging nettles he would have the best possible natural 'injection'.

He set about mixing homoeopathic calcium with the extract of the stinging nettle and discovered a very good end product, which for hot flushes can be very important and can reduce their frequency and intensity. During hot flushes there is a rapid decrease of oestrogen and exacerbating that with bad dietary habits, or by drinking or smoking, will influence the situation detrimentally. It is even worse when women in the menopause become uninterested in food. They become thin and sometimes almost anorexic, and the symptoms will go from bad to worse. The secret is to keep head and hands cool, and often it is better to eat smaller meals, but perhaps increase the number of meals taken during the day.

There are several positive steps a woman can take that will pay off. My wife keeps busier than ever and she remains interested in life, in the family and what is happening in the world. Do not hide behind the excuse of having to get through the menopause first, and after that everything will fall into place. Ignore the symptoms as much as possible and the hot flushes will soon reduce naturally and spontaneously. Sometimes women choose to take an oestrogen supplement to bring the problem under control quickly, but the bad news is that the hot flushes will return with more severity as soon as that drug is discontinued. Therefore it is important to look for natural treatment, for example some of the water treatments, which are described in my book *Water – Healer or Poison?*

Another excellent remedy is the Menopausal Formula from Dr Vogel, designed to control depression, hot flushes, hysteria, headaches, irritability and nervous exhaustion. A vitamin E supplement can also help. There are other positive steps one can take, such as energy balancing. Aromatherapy or reflexology can also be successful contributors to the relief of hot flushes, and more information about such methods can be found in my book *Body Energy*. These sudden and intense episodes of heat usually come without warning or pattern. Mostly the heat starts in the chest, neck or face, and then radiates all over the body. I have often been able to help patients by recommending vitamin E or bioflavenoids. It can be helpful to use vitamin E in combination with ginseng, as this will boost the production and supply of natural oestrogen and so give considerable relief from hot flushes and associated conditions.

Some women exaggerate the incidence of hot flushes in a plea for attention and sympathy from their partner. It should be understood that hot flushes will happen long before the actual menopause and may gradually increase in severity. Fortunately not all women experience these to the same troublesome intensity. However, I can well understand that if nothing is done to ease the situation, these hot flushes can be extremely embarrassing and bothersome. One lady described them to me as follows: 'My blood is boiling and I feel on fire. My hair is wet and I cannot sleep and sometimes I lie awake all night bathed in sweat.' I told her not to despair and prescribed Salvia, Urticalcin, a vitamin E supplement and Optivite. Later she wrote to me that her hot flushes were very much less troublesome and also that she had long spells where she had no problems at all.

No two women are alike in the way they experience the menopause. Some women may suffer from hot flushes for days on end; others may just experience the odd hot flush, lasting no longer than a few minutes. The length of time during which these symptoms occur varies greatly, because the menopause can take anything from one year to six years. Unlike some other menopausal problems, research results indicate that the majority of women (from 70 to 90 per cent) experience hot flushes and this makes it the most frequently experienced menopausal symptom. Nobody really knows what signals are emitted by the body, although it is certain that the oestrogen levels are decreasing while the FSH levels increase in women who suffer from hot flushes. It is indeed very often a matter of taking a positive attitude and setting about helping oneself. Always try to be relaxed about the situation and do not fret or worry, because one thing is certain: they will pass. Relaxation exercises, acupuncture or cranial osteopathy may be of help. Whatever your individual experiences or symptoms, do not give in to them, because help is always available. Always look on the bright side and remember that they are temporary. They will disappear in the same way they sneaked up on you. One day you'll suddenly realise that you haven't had a hot flush for quite some time and you won't even have missed them.

Chapter 4

Osteoporosis

OSTEOPOROSIS IS A thinning of the bones involving a gradual reduction in the bone mass, so that the skeleton becomes weakened. Even in pre-menopausal conditions up to five per cent of bone mass can be lost.

In recent years it seems to be that this problem is getting worse. During the thirty-odd years I have been in practice I have treated many patients for back or neck problems, but recently it seems that there are more than ever. It worries me greatly when I see a patient and yet I know that I can no longer relieve his or her symptoms by manipulation. Their bones have become too brittle and it is indeed a great worry to any osteopath or chiropractor to deal with these bone structures confidently. This is then one further reason why I always insist that patients ensure that they select an experienced and well-qualified practitioner, or much damage can be inflicted. It is very hard for a practitioner to refuse treatment when the patient pleads for him to apply manipulation and begs to be relieved from the pain and discomfort. However, sometimes the risk is just not justified. To understand a little about the human frame and the bone structure, one must realise that bones do not move of their own volition. It is the muscles that move the bones. Sometimes it is extremely dangerous, when the muscles have grown weak and the bones have become porotic, to apply manipulation. This means that, wherever possible, other forms of treatment, especially those aimed at early prevention, should be explored.

During different phases in one's life the skeleton loses bone density. Both men and women start to lose calcium from their bones from the age of about 35 onwards. After the menopause, some women (but not all) seem to lose it more quickly as the oestrogen level drops. The effect of this may not show up until the seventies when brittle bones then become noticeable. Only 20–30 per cent of older women show any obvious sign of this condition. You may have enough natural oestrogen after the menopause to stop the rapid loss of calcium. But the condition is often made worse by smoking and heavy drinking, lack of exercise and lack of sunshine, as well as by a poor diet low in calcium. You can help yourself to keep brittle bones at bay by adopting a healthy diet and making sure of sufficient exercise.

There are certain clearly identified factors indicating a higher risk of contracting osteoporosis. One is to be female. There can also be a family history of the condition. Other factors include liver disease, smoking, drinking, anorexia or bulimia nervosa. However, during the menopause women are more vulnerable to this problem than at any other stage of their life.

When I mention the endocrine system, I am often tempted to draw the analogy with a musical orchestra. When the thyroid gland, one of the major endocrine glands, is out of tune, this can be a contributory factor towards the development of an osteoporitic condition. With arthritics or bronchial patients, or people who are on long-term steroid treatment, one must remain on the alert for this condition. And let's not be blinkered and think that this condition is reserved only for the older generation, because even at a younger age the damage can be telling. I remember a young girl who was in agony because of a back problem. I diagnosed clear signs of osteoporosis and therefore I was unable to help her with manipulation, and had to look to other ways to help her. Contrary to popular belief, even hormone replacement therapy does not always have the answer. We must always keep an open mind and continue to explore other solutions.

If there is evidence of a family history of osteoporosis and the loss of bone mass appears to be genetical, drastic steps are called for to overcome this problem. On the basis of statistics gathered in the USA and the UK, it is thought that one in four women will experience health problems related to osteoporosis. These may take the form of fractures, or sometimes multiple fractures, in the hip, wrist, or in the dorsal spine. From statistics it appears that each year 45,000 hip fractures occur in women over the age of 65 (around 17 per cent of women in this age group). Often I have been asked to treat patients who have had a vertebral crush or a dowager hump. This is a classic example of the thinning bones syndrome. As time goes on this problem gets worse and if there is real concern about a hereditary factor being involved, one is fully justified in demanding an X-ray or a bone scan. These tests may indeed be helpful to diagnose the symptoms at an early stage.

Women approaching the age of 40 are at the highest risk of loss of bone mass: from that age onwards, the loss is likely to be a minimum of one per cent per year at a conservative estimate. After the menopause bone loss increases and a further 10 to 15 years on the bone density will have changed very considerably. Because of this rapid decrease, many elderly women will experience a fracture one way or another. By taking some early precautions much can be done to help oneself. I have already mentioned the value of Urticalcin, but comfrey is also of great benefit. According to one's individual preference this can be used in tablet form or by drinking comfrey tea. Hemp nettle extract, or Galeopsis is also a recommended means of maintaining one's calcium level. However, nutrition is most important and in a later chapter I will give some more detailed advice on this subject.

In all medical conditions circulation is important because effective elimination is needed to maintain good health. When the consciousness of the nervous system is confused by our misunderstanding of physical ailments and our anatomy, the circulation of the blood is impeded. Quite rightly we worry about high or low blood pressure, and these conditions are responsible for defective elimination.

Good posture contributes to healthy circulation, although on the whole we pay little attention to posture. If the framework or skeleton is in the correct position, the nerves, arteries and veins are free, enabling efficient circulation of the blood to all parts of the body, allowing the nerves to function properly.

The first steps towards attaining correct posture is to pay attention to the neck and shoulders, remembering that if the neck is crooked and the shoulders are out of alignment, the position of the internal organs is likely to be affected. The shoulder blades are responsible for the condition of the neck. If your right shoulder is lower and appears to be longer than the left, you will find the left shoulder blade to be an inch higher than the right. When examining the back of the shoulder, you will feel a large solid lump. If the right shoulder blade has moved down, there is very little tension, if any, above the shoulder blade. The right shoulder blade will push the spine out of position to the left, or move closer to the left shoulder blade. This causes the seventh cervical vertebra (the large bone on the back of the neck) to move to the left. The cervical region, or bones of the neck, will draw to the right and cause the atlas or top bone of the neck to twist out of position.

By closely examining the front of your neck, you may find that the right side of your neck seems to be a little larger and firmer. This is the starting point for trouble with the eyes, ears, nose and mouth, and migraine headaches. Your chest will become prominent, or fuller on the left side, while on the right side a depression will be noticed, which will interfere with your breathing. Such cases are termed tuberculosis of the lungs. The reverse condition of the chest would indicate a wheezing or asthma.

I would imagine that it is obvious that when one stands with the left shoulder lowered, the spine will move to a different position. Again, when the left shoulder is raised, the opposite shoulder drops. This gives a quick and clear understanding of how the spine moves from a certain position and how rigid the ligaments become inside the body under the higher shoulder. Consequently the opposite side becomes relaxed and forces the internal organs of the body to move out of place and become congested.

The mineral calcium fluoride will help osteoporosis patients as it strengthens the tissues of the 'conscious system', so that our understanding may be strong and alert. It builds within our body, bone, brain and consciousness, the faculty of understanding. The less of this mineral we possess, the slower our understanding becomes.

Calcium fluoride is yellowish-green in colour. It is used extensively and therefore if the strength of this mineral in the body decreases, it needs to be replaced. Fortunately it is possible to replenish this in natural ways. The mineral travels from the adenoids to the mid-brain, from where it is directed to the cell tissue, reaching every part of the conscious system. Calcium fluoride is used especially in the treatment of the brain, bones, the conscious system, the sinuses, the teeth, the adenoids, the stomach and bowels, and the pituitary and pineal glands.

Next, we should realise that each organ of our body, as well as the skin, must be replenished with fresh mineral as it becomes exhausted; in the same way as we replenish our store cupboard – which the grocer does for us.

We are particular that our personal appearance is exactly as it should be. We are interested in our face, hair and our dress. Our necktie must be perfectly knotted and in position, and our shoes shined. We assume the best possible attitude towards our customers or clients in order to make a good impression necessary to gain their respect and trust. To present ourselves in the best possible light, our approach must be perfect. We smile and express a friendly interest and approach, but from the outset we must be certain that our attire is properly arranged. This gives us the self-confidence we need. To achieve all this we pay attention to detail. For example, we bathe and use deodorant and perfume or aftershave, and wear freshly laundered and ironed clothes. We make sure that our nails are clean and properly shaped. In short, we make sure that physically we pass the first inspection with flying colours. There is just one minor thing that always seems to be overlooked, mainly because it is not immediately noticeable – we have forgotten to check that we are internally clean and well-groomed too. This is when diet is so important.

We often fall short of the things we wish to accomplish. With a sick and ailing body we are unable to do many of those things we would so much like to do and attain the look and shape we most admire. We can take care of our exterior with soap and water, cosmetics, etc. Yet, we forget that we are able to achieve the same results and cleanliness for the interior – with correct dietary management. Once our bodies have been cleansed on the inside, the outside will not need any cosmetics.

It's easy to believe, because of the link between menopausal osteoporosis and oestrogen deficiencies, that a hormonal supplement can successfully treat this condition. Often it is also considered to be a sensible preventative measure. Alas, I have already mentioned that this is not the natural way and there is always a slightly increased risk of breast cancer. Why not then consider some dietary change, including the use of supplementary vitamins, minerals and trace elements and a bona fide calcium supplement?

If we have aches and pains in the back or the limbs, shortening of the spine or even severe pain in the surrounding area of the back, it is sensible to take note and see what can be done to improve the situation. In the case of an osteoporotic condition we must see that the posture is correct, i.e. sitting and walking with a straight back and shoulders down, and avoiding the carrying of heavy loads. This is especially important for elderly people. General dietary advice is to eat raw, dark-green vegetables, sesame seeds, kelp, carrots, berries and fruit, etc. Chronic osteoporosis can cause pains in the legs, excessive hair growth, dryness or vaginal itching and other unpleasant symptoms. Both for younger and elderly people with osteoporosis I must emphasise that careful exercise is necessary, but for the elderly generation especially I would suggest that they choose gentle ways of exercising. I cannot help but repeat the all-important message: 'Prevention is better than cure' and, given that the problem of osteoporosis nowadays is more wide spread, it is important to take some early preventative measures rather than allowing this disabling condition to fully develop before deciding to do something about it. People who are inactive, confined to a chair or bed, lose the calcium from their bones much more quickly, while people who use their limbs in a more active manner, e.g. walking, cycling or swimming, arrest or slow down the degeneration.

My final advice to osteoporosis patients is to use a good vitamin and mineral balancer. Nature's Best makes a preparation called Osteo-Balance and in the accompanying literature the manufacturer stresses the fact that most people know that calcium is needed for healthy bones. Recent research has spread uncertainty about the theory that taking extra calcium is the ready answer. Indeed, the practice has become popular with post-menopausal women who seek to maintain bone strength and other people with special calcium needs, but it is a fact that scientists have discovered that magnesium may be equally if not more important than calcium. The conclusion is that a combination of these two major minerals may be of most benefit. The concern is over the release of the two hormones that control calcium's fate. If the calcium is left to circulate in the blood or to be excreted in high levels in the urine – rather than laid down as bones – it can accumulate and harden arteries, or turn up as kidney stones. All research concludes that what is needed is the right balance of calcium and magnesium, along with the correct amounts of vitamin D to maintain absorption. Nature's Best Osteo-Balance has been developed, bearing in mind the need for acid/alkaline balance in the stomach and contains a span of special forms of calcium – citrate, carbonate, lactate and gluconate – to give the best possible chance of absorption. Each Osteo-Balance capsule provides:

Calcium citrate	63mg
Calcium gluconate	48mg
Calcium lactate	28mg
Calcium orotate	28mg
Calcium carbonate	18mg
(Equivalent to 33 mg of elemental calcium)	
Magnesium L-aspartate	205mg
Magnesium thiosulphate	123mg
Magnesium orotate	82mg
(Equivalent to 33mg of elemental magnesium)	
Vitamin D_3	50iu

It has been my intention to give osteoporotic readers hope and to inform them that there are plenty of ways to avoid harsh or unnatural treatment. Carefully consider the indications and symptoms, or messages emitted by the body, and plan your strategy accordingly.

In further chapters I will deal with other symptoms or messages, where, again, the same principle applies: if these messages are interpreted correctly, much misery can be avoided.

Chapter 5

Restless Legs

FEMALE PATIENTS APPROACHING the menopause often complain that they cannot sleep or relax because of an uncontrollable restlessness or irritability in their legs. When lying in bed they cannot bear to have their legs covered by bedclothes and are compelled to have them sticking out at the side. They have involuntary urges to kick out as they feel a sudden fidgety jumpiness in their lower limbs.

I must say that this feeling is not a symptom that is especially significant of the menopause. At any time it is a message from the circulatory system that something ought to be done, before it develops into a more difficult and permanent situation with far-reaching problems. Although the circulatory system undergoes a major change during the menopause, restless legs are not only due to hormonal changes; they can also be the result of a mineral deficiency. This creepy sensation is felt deep inside the legs and often occurs while relaxing in the evening or night, when one becomes fidgety and uncomfortable for no obvious reason. Although there is really no known cause for this, we know that it is mostly of circulatory origin, and that a vitamin E supplement will help. Walking, massaging or rubbing the legs will also bring relief.

Studies have shown why a deficiency of vitamin E may cause leg cramps, and the effects are more pronounced at the menopausal stage, when the hormone system has temporarily lost its balance. In the case of a deficiency of vitamin E there is a definite progressive loss of muscular co-ordination and reflexes, a loss of sensation in the peripheral nerves and an involvement of the spinal cord. It is often noticed that poor fat absorption coincides with extremely low blood and tissue levels of vitamin E. The reason for the deficiency does not fall into any of the categories that can be explained. Often there does not appear to be an unusual destruction of vitamin E by some other compound in the body, nor is there any underlying problem with absorption. We can be sure of one thing; that if we respond by supplementing with fat-soluble vitamin E (even with levels that overload the system) the body is unable to absorb this. Most likely this is because the liver is not doing its job properly. However, it is possible to correct this deficiency with water-soluble vitamin E. Sometimes it is beneficial to use a combination of the vitamins E and C. Research has indicated that vitamin C boosts the immune system and aids the body's defence against infectious diseases. Vitamin E also acts as an anti-oxidant, which means that it protects cells and tissue from gradual deterioration caused by excessive oxidation. In principle this is the same process that occurs when butter turns rancid or fruit turns brown. So the anti-oxidant protection is also of importance and it is widely believed that vitamin E is a tremendous help for restless legs.

Vitamin E is the most powerful vitamin part of the body's anti-oxidant defence system. It is the prime agent that prevents fatty acids from reacting with oxygen to form harmful toxins, known as lipid peroxides. Not only does vitamin E protect fats in the body, but other vital nutrients such as vitamin A, the B-complex vitamins and vitamin C are also protected.

Anti-oxidant vitamin E allows the more efficient use of oxygen by the blood and muscles, so it is favoured by sports people who are working to increase their stamina and endurance by training the heart and circulatory system. Vitamin E is necessary for the health of the reproductive system, the integrity of red blood cells and for the functioning of the white blood cells of the immune system. Nature's Best d alpha tocopherol is 36 per cent more potent than the synthetic dL form, weight for weight, and is derived completely from soyabeans.

As explained, restless legs can be due to a slightly impaired circulatory system, but there can also be a possible tissue weakening, and therefore we must look at ways of strengthening the muscles. The stronger the muscles, the better the circulation and the fewer problems there are with restless legs and cramps. In this respect it is sometimes helpful to supplement iron. This mineral controls the health of the flesh of the entire body, including the muscles.

When the term 'muscles' is used, we don't realise what an extensive network of muscle and fibrous tissues covers our body. There are muscles that are connected to the cartilage in the joints of our body. Whenever the flesh connects with this so-called 'elastic fibre' it acts as a muscle. Our entire body contains muscles and without them movement would be impossible. We have muscles from the top of our head, right down to our toes. First, we have the scalp muscles that cause the scalp to move forward and backward, followed by the muscles over the eyes that allow us to move our forehead up and down. Then we have the muscles of the ears, eyes and nostrils. The outer muscles of the face surround the mouth and the eyes, extending from one to the other. Leaving our chin, the muscles travel down to the collar bone, and the back of the head. The muscles leave the mastoid glands and travel down into the interior of the body. In other words, the muscles of the face alone form an ingenious and intricate network.

Beneath the skin, there are three layers of flesh. Muscles are connected to each one of these layers, and also to all parts of the skin. There are muscles in our chest and muscles of a fleshy disposition leaving each rib, connecting the ribs together and extending through the entire thorax and diaphragm. From the different ribs, the muscles connect with the sacrum where they take on a different shape and travel down into the feet. The largest and arguably most important muscle is in the calf of the leg. There are also muscles in each of our toes.

Turning back to the upper part of the body, there are also muscles in the tongue, the larynx and pharynx, the stomach, bowels, heart and lungs, not forgetting that the liver and gall-bladder are also equipped with a set of muscles. From the shoulders, muscles run down the arms to the hands. Every joint of our skeleton is controlled by muscles. At some point the fibrous tissue attaches itself to the bone. There are also muscles in the intestines, colon and rectum, as well as in the anus, sphincter, kidneys and urinary organs. Although we are usually only aware of a few muscles (such as those in the eyes, throat, tongue and heart), the body contains hundreds of muscles making up the greater part of its fleshy area. Iron will provide strength to all these different muscles of the body.

Some of the muscles belong to the voluntary system and the spine. The muscles of this system comprise fibrous tissue surrounding the skeleton and connecting with the nervous system. They are distinct from the muscles of the involuntary nervous system. Other groups are the muscles of the flesh and skin.

We are aware of important muscles – like those causing the blinking of the eyes or the movement of various parts of our body – because they are composed of delicate tissue, as are other muscles, such as those in the tonsils, the larynx and the pharynx. Each time our throat is sore, understand that all these muscles are impaired and must be treated. Each and every muscle has its part to play.

Just visualise the amount of muscular fibre connected with the lymphatic system and the arteries. Every node and bypass in the lymphatic system is provided with muscle, and as the lymph passes into these different glands, the action of the muscles opens and closes the small lobes. The same applies to the muscle in our arteries and veins. They are of much greater importance than some of the better-known muscles. Of course, when asked to name some muscles, those of our arms are the first we think of, followed by the muscles in the calves of our legs. But all the soreness that is caused in the body, hips and legs is due to muscular impairment in the loins or the lumbar region – in other words in the small of the back. The same applies to the ovarian gland, the fallopian tubes, and the uterine and vaginal muscles. Taking all of this into consideration, the mineral iron performs an important function in keeping all these muscles in working strength. Moreover it also maintains the skin so that it may carry on its own activity.

Let's go back for a moment to the complicated group of organs that are connected to the sacral-plexus. These include the bladder, the uterus, the ovaries, the prostate gland, the testicles and, below the hip bones, the rectum. When the muscles of the pelvis are disconnected, it causes trouble for these organs. Whenever the vitality and strength are cut off, the framework of the back must be corrected, so that strength can be rebuilt in every part of the body that has grown weak.

If the muscles of the urinary organs have weakened, strength must be restored to the different parts of these organs. The crucial location is in the small of the back, just above the hips at approximately the fourth and fifth lumbar vertebrae. In the female the uterine organs, the fallopian tubes, the ovaries and the uterus are also treated from this position of the body. By placing the hand on the area covering the break between the lowest lumbar vertebra and the sacrum, a reflex will travel down through the muscles on the left into the feet. The area of the sacrum, just above the coccyx connects with the muscles of the rectum and the anus, muscles which need to be strong and healthy in order to perform their daily duty. Irritation and constipation arise from a weakness in this part of the body. The area of the third and fourth lumbar vertebrae connects with the muscles of the colon and the rectum. By now you may have come to realise that individual sections of the spine relate to various organs or parts of the body. At this point I will not go into any further detail because it is not relevant to the menopause but it was my intention to emphasise the intricacies of the muscular system and the essential need to maintain it in good order. Adequate supplies of iron will help a great deal in this direction. Since the heart consists of muscular tissue, iron is essential for its maintenance and this applies to all the organs and muscles in the body.

The reason why I have gone into considerable detail here is not only because restless legs are a fairly common complaint, but also because there are so many theories regarding it. Unfortunately it is often noted as 'cause unknown'.

The most widely accepted diagnosis of restless legs is that it is a circulatory problem. Blood provides the motor power of the body; without this motor power it is impossible to move a leg or raise an arm until the force of blood first penetrates that portion of the body. Take for instance a paralytic or arthritic case, where circulation to the limbs has been severely reduced and the patient is unable to move the affected limb. Why? Not only because of nerve damage, but also because there is insufficient blood in those parts to furnish the motor power.

Blood is made up of fluids containing blood cells. It is pumped throughout the body by the heart, passing from the arteries into the veins. The food that we eat stimulates the blood to a certain extent and when the nutrients of the food combine with the white and red cells and nourish the tissue, the tissue becomes stronger and gives us more vitality. When the veins and arteries are free from pressure the blood circulates freely. As it passes to the lungs, heat is transferred to the iron molecules, spreading warmth and vitality to every part of the body.

At normal blood pressure it should take three minutes for a unit of blood to leave the heart, make a complete revolution of the body and return to the lungs. Ease of this circulation is of the utmost importance. The large veins on the outer part of our body are not as easily congested as the ones in the deep part of the flesh. The more congestion in the flesh, the harder and more congested the body becomes and the more pressure is raised in the inner circulation. This causes the body to become cold and sluggish. The lack of heat in the blood prevents the hormones from working naturally. To use an analogy, the circulation of red blood resembles a hot water system. It is supposed to furnish heat to all parts of our body, which will allow the digestive juices to flow freely, giving correct action to the digestive tract and the elimination process.

We should never allow the pulse to become low or irregular. By keeping track of our pulse it is possible to detect problems at an early stage. If the pulse appears to be fast and jerky, it means that circulation in the spine, shoulders, neck, arms and legs is defective.

The heart is a pump composed of muscles, fibrous tissue and elastic fibre. In order to stimulate the function of this vital organ Dr Vogel has devised an excellent remedy which I have often prescribed for circulatory problems, and especially for restless legs. This remedy is called Hyperisan and is specially designed to strengthen the veins, promote circulation and prevent brittleness of the capillaries. It contains yarrow, horse chestnut, St John's wort and arnica, and, together with a vitamin E supplement and Urticalcin, I have found it a most effective treatment to overcome restless legs.

Time and again, some of the components of the herbal kingdom still manage to amaze me. For years, like many others, I used to regard herbs from a scientific viewpoint, but latterly I look for specific characteristics; in other words the individual signature of all that grows. Similarities to health problems or minor weaknesses in the body often give us clear signs as to which plant we should use for treatment. I remember meeting an old lady when I visited the Shetland Isles, quite some time ago now. She spoke about St John's wort (*Hypericum perforatum*) with something akin to devotion. Whenever possible, I like to learn from the elderly generation, especially when they live in isolated places, about how they used to treat health problems when a doctor wasn't available. Many of them have told me about interesting natural ways of treatment, knowledge of which has been passed on to them by their forebears. This lady explained that *Hypericum* contains a message, and the easy way to recognise this message is by steeping the herb in water or oil. It will then turn a deep red colour and this characteristic clearly shows that *Hypericum* should be used for the treatment of blood disorders. Considering *Hypericum perforatum* in its full beauty, it is possible to pharmacologically or scientifically find an explanation for some of these claims, but secondly we should then look at the information received by looking at the plant. Every living thing has significance. Very often the name of the herb or plant indicates some specific property and in the case of *Hypericum*, the common name of St John's wort proves this philosophy. The leaves, with their tiny oil glands, look as if they have been perforated, which explains the Latin name. The oil they contain is a deep blood-red colour and not only does it work very effectively to enhance circulation of the blood, but it also serves as a natural tranquilliser. One of my oldest friends, Dr Hans Moolenburgh, believes that the name St John (peace giver and lover of mankind – one of the best loved apostles in the scriptures) denotes the plant's peace-giving properties. Restless legs are a symbol that the body is not at peace, and when this is the case, possibly because of menstrual circumstances, or perhaps depression because of an inner crisis, this remedy will help in an exceptional way.

The more I study natural medicine, the better I learn to interpret the messages supplied by nature to the advantage of our health. Quite often it is impossible to explain these messages scientifically and yet in their characteristics there can be found a plea to be used for a specific purpose. Rarely have I received what I consider to be a correct answer when I have asked medical students for an explanation of science. My favourite interpretation, which I found in one of my dictionaries, is 'Science is the discovery of the secrets of nature and the process by which they are made available for the benefit of mankind.'

Chapter 6

Depression

THIS MORNING, determined to start the chapter on the subject of depression, I temporarily submitted to temptation and had a brisk walk first. Today is a typical example of a glorious autumn day; the sun is shining and my eyes are drawn to the garden beyond the window where I can see the beautiful colours of fallen and falling leaves. Yesterday it was raining and everything outside looked grim. Today, with the sun shining, the world looks beautiful. Speaking personally, autumn is never my favourite season, because it reminds me of the end of summer. While preparing this chapter I was reminded of the many patients I have treated over the years who are of the same opinion. When asked to analyse their emotions, many of them described a feeling that life had ended. Our common sense tells us that this is only partly true, because spring and summer will return after the winter season. Moreover, the winter season is not a time of death, but of new beginnings. It has its own attractions of bracing frost and beautiful white snow. Despite the cold, growth continues, albeit rarely visible. I have often pointed this out to my patients who felt as if life had ended. Winter is actually more like a beginning. With the wisdom life has brought, we must not dwell on what has passed, but look forward to what lies ahead. Think of what nature has brought us and will bring again. Unfortunately, too often I have seen that depression has been allowed to rule or ruin someone's life.

Recently I was asked for help by a charming middle-aged lady who was in the depths of depression. As sometimes happens at this stage of a woman's life, her sexual needs and appetite had diminished and her husband, lacking understanding of her physiological changes, had found himself a younger woman. He had told his wife that the new woman in his life was the perfect match for him and much more attractive. Very possibly he will soon realise that he has made a major mistake. There is so much more to life if it has been shared with the same partner for a long time. The memories of those years cannot be enjoyed or shared with anyone else. Even the memories of the children, of specific instances or events relating to their parents, will be different from their parents' memories. Losing a partner often causes emotional poverty, especially if it has been a close and long-term relationship. This lady had good reason to be disappointed and during the autumn season especially such emotions can easily get out of hand. I did stress that she should look forward to another future, because she would be the winner. Not only mentally will she be a better and more understanding person, she will also be able to understand her children better when they grow older. If a relationship cannot be mended it is probably better to bring it to an end, so that there is the hope of a better relationship some time in the future.

So often I hear people expressing the fear that at 50 life is over for them and they dare not look forward to another fulfilling relationship. Fortunately I have also often heard about happy new beginnings. The state of mind is crucial and we must always believe that we become stronger because of our experiences. There is some truth in the old saying: 'If we please ourselves, we weaken ourselves and others.' So, for the formation of our personality it is important that we stand up and face the trials of life. Living in the past must be replaced by positive thoughts for the future. Such a positive mental approach goes hand-in-hand with our physical well-being, because strength and durability are required in every aspect of our daily physical existence.

In trying to establish this positive attitude in our body, brain and consciousness, it is important to develop a strong character since this forms the most important balance in material life. If our character is strengthened to the point of firmness, it is easy to resist or overcome temptation and our body is in a condition to ward off sickness and pain. As soon as our character becomes better balanced, we will start to provide strength for our entire system. This keeps the nerves from atrophying which causes so much damage to our bodies. When the nerves are well balanced, we become free from kidney disturbances and our urinary system becomes strong and in good working condition. Strength in the tissues of the creative organs overcomes ovarian trouble, slackness of the uterus, and helps the sacral plexus to work properly and actively in its connection with the different organs in this part of the body.

Worry, fear and unnatural desires are caused by a lack of strength in our brain and in our nerves. If we wish to be free from jealousy and unhealthy desire, there must be strength of will and character. How true it is that after each spell of sickness our friends say: 'Well, as soon as you regain your strength, you will be all right.' But how will we regain our strength when the circulation of our blood has been impaired, causing a lack of strength in every part of our body? After each attack of so-called 'sickness' – no matter how great or small – the vitality of the body is diminished. This will probably affect the posture and position of the neck. Next, we'll discover a weakness in the small of our back, from where it will travel to the hips and lower limbs, most likely causing congestion and settling in our feet.

People who have depleted their strength through worry and depression find that their back is sore until it seems almost impossible to follow their daily routine. Sometimes the lack of strength from worry can cause such misery that even getting up out of a chair can become a painful effort.

It becomes easier to control one's emotions if the mineral content of the body is well balanced. Posture is also important: watch the shoulders, neck and arms and see that they are straight and free from impingements, especially the lower part of the back, the short ribs (lumbars), hips and the pelvic bone. If this is not the case see that it is remedied. By ensuring that our frame is erect and sufficient minerals are flowing through the body, all ovarian, uterine and menstrual troubles will diminish or be overcome.

Man's body is a peculiar, but perfect, structure. We find as many bones and joints in our feet as there are in our spine, from the atlas at the top, to the lower end of the coccyx. The spinal cord, with its various nerve branches, supplies nerve impulses to all the different parts of the body, if the posture allows. Remember that blood is essential for life. In turn, the blood supply is dependent upon the body's network of glands, each set of glands secreting different substances into the bloodstream. The importance of the glands should never be overlooked.

There is another very important factor and that is the will: the will to do something, and to do it well. While growing up I remember my mother always telling us '*cannot* is lying in the cemetery next to *will not*'. The will to overcome problems can be enhanced and encouraged by natural means. I have already mentioned calcium, which is important for the treatment of depression, as well as several other remedies. Let me remind you that calcium rebuilds the bone and supplies strong determination or willpower to the body, brain and consciousness of man. It nourishes the will to discount and overcome any infirmity or ailment. When the calcium level in the body is low, the will is weak and one tends to submit to impulses that are often regretted later. Weakness of the body caused by a deficient calcium level is a further reason why we allow so many wonderful opportunities to pass by without taking advantage of them.

It helps to understand the difference between the divine will and the physical will. Our emotions are controlled by the physical will. Divine will separates right from wrong, making our existence happier. The two wills working in harmony enable us to set in motion any of the organs of our body, overcoming such troubles as a sluggish, torpid liver, or a stomach or bowel disorder, and will justly regulate all our internal workings.

The will is one of the most essential functions in man. It has a tendency to predominate over all other functions, but when properly controlled it contributes to harmony between other functions as well as both physical and spiritual strength. Egotism is not will; neither is determination. Both egotism and determination, however, are the baser instincts that destroy will and also the physical body.

If you believe yourself to be under the control of another person's will, and if you allow this to continue, the result will be that your own will is gradually eroded. If you continue to submit to the domination of another, you will finally lose control of your own life.

Will is a very important part of man's nature. It provides power to move or remain still, and, according to the amount of calcium that the system contains, one can cause the body, brain and consciousness to obey each command. It gives us the power of control over habits of all kinds, especially those which we desire to overcome.

Calcium is essential to the bones, the muscles, the nerves and fibrous tissues of our body. Without the power of will, our existence becomes despondent and listless, and trouble will appear in many different parts of the body – a sore neck, painful and tired shoulders and arms, backache, or trouble in the knees, the ankles or in the feet and metatarsal arches. A lack of calcium in the elastic fibre will allow the bones of the skull and the face to move out of position, causing sinus trouble and eye strain.

There is no need to undergo complicated tests to determine the amount of calcium your system requires. We do many things that we do not wish to. Later we say 'oh, I wish I could have refused, I wish I had said no'. Our attitude shows a lack of resistance, which is a lack of will. That lack of will is caused by a calcium deficiency in our system. When the calcium level is replenished and properly distributed, we have much less trouble in conducting our affairs to suit ourselves. It will be just as easy to refuse as it will to accept. A supplementary calcium preparation will re-establish our will and calcium absorbed by the tissues of the body will, in turn, create a new body, brain and consciousness.

If we stand on the bank of a river and watch the water flowing down its course, we notice small stones or pebbles gathering moss day by day. Each pebble, each stone will gather moss until it has reached the point where it can hold no more. The excess moss, and more, will break away, and continue to be transported down the creek until it finds another object to cling to. The body, like the pebble gathering moss, receives fresh supplies of calcium which cause the decomposed mineral matter to break away to be eliminated from our body through its natural channel. The decomposed mineral passes into the red blood, into the veins, then into the ventricles, and on to the kidneys where filtering takes place. From there it is eliminated through the urinary organs. This process continues until the power of will is re-established, giving us new strength to overcome all obstacles in our path and establish new management, new life, and a new outlook, and an entire new existence, which helps towards a happy and contented life.

Understand that the will acts in many different ways. It affects our mental state and our conscious system. Materially, it acts on the bony structure of our body. The first consideration should be the skull and its elastic fibre. Next we should have the calcium restored to our neck, shoulders and arms, and make sure that the spine has plenty of calcium, from the atlas to the coccyx. The ribs are also important as nerves extend from our spine along the ribs to different parts of our body. If we have a crooked skeleton, it will interfere with moisture in the joints and the coccyx, resulting in impaired circulation through these areas.

Each part of our body must have sufficient calcium to enable the conscious system to perform without interference. Calcium is necessary for the skeleton, the brain, the involuntary nervous system, the hair, and for the finger- and toenails. The blood must also have its share of calcium.

When most of our wrongdoings occur, we are aware of the consequences, but as our will is weakened and our system below par, caused by the lack of calcium, we do not have the power to resist the wrong we are about to do. For example, there are many very fine people who have one fault: the indulgence of alcohol. They become intoxicated and do and say rash things they would not consider doing or saying when sober. The will has been weakened and there is no resistance in the body or mind. When the right level of calcium and ferrum phosphate is established in such individuals, the habit of drinking alcohol disappears without craving.

Of course mankind is inhibited by so many external influences that more often than not no real effort is made to gain control of the impulses that run loose in the world. It always has been, and still is, easier to let things go on as they are, rather than exert the will to change them.

We are all creatures of emotions, passions, circumstances and accident. States of the mind, heart and body are shaped by the drift of life, even when special attention is given to any of them. If you take time to contemplate for a while, you will be surprised to find how much of your life has been mere drift; how little you have done towards investigating the power that operates in animal volition, from where it originates, how it is controlled and how it may be utilised.

Any created form of life is worth studying to see the effort of self-expression. A tree sends its branches towards the sunlight, while through its roots it struggles in a search for water. This is what is called inanimate life, but it represents a force that comes from some source and continues to equilibrium.

Mankind is a higher form of life than animal, and animal life is above the level of vegetation. There are more millions of flesh cells in the body than our mind could conceive. Every single one of these cells originated in vegetable form, but it could not have originated without some force that existed in and of the cell itself.

I would suggest calling this force energy, but you are free to give it any scientific name you please. It has been called by various names in different studies, but the terms used do not help the average person to understand it any better. It is often the case that when a new book is written the author believes that his invention of some new scientific word may establish a new science and draw all students to his feet. Once in a while a simple word is sufficient to explain a new idea, but the disposition of scientific writers to invent hundreds of long technical terms has made their special literature inaccessible for the majority of readers.

There is no place on the globe where energy is not found. The air is so loaded with it that in the cold north, the sky shines in boreal rays – and wherever the frigid temperature yields to warmth the electrical conditions can cause alarm. Water is nominally a liquid union of gases but it is charged with electrical, mechanical and chemical energies, any one of which is capable of doing great service as well as great damage to man. Even ice, in its coldest phase, has energy, for it is not subdued, nor even still. Its force has broken mountain rocks into fragments, and the person who has suffered from depression may be able to relate to that. He or she may have felt at times like a rock that has become fragmented and all purpose in life has disappeared.

The nervous system is very intricate. It can easily be disturbed, even by a very minor vibration, when it can shatter. Some while ago I was consulted by a woman of about 30 who was convinced that she was in the first throes of the menopause. I told her that her age and symptoms did not relate, but she insisted that she had read up on the subject and several of her friends, to whom she had described her symptoms, had also told her that it must be the menopause. She was thoroughly depressed and had allowed her nervous system to deteriorate so badly that she couldn't sleep: the analogy of a fragmented rock certainly appeared fitting. She claimed that she had no energy, no future to look forward to any more, and it may all be just as well over and done with. That was the state of her mind. I feel utterly sad when I hear a person so thoroughly depressed and without hope. I decided to give her acupuncture treatment and some natural remedies and indeed we managed to reverse the situation. It just goes to show that the nervous system is a major factor, both mentally and physically. Lack of determination causes a weakness of the nervous system, throwing the whole body out of balance. The atlas, or top bone of the spine, can become dislodged, even only fractionally, causing a ringing and itching of the ears. A weakness of the nervous system affects the eyes, causing poor sight and twitching of the muscles, and can easily affect the stomach and bowels.

All ailments or infirmities are due partly to poor circulation and partly to a nervous condition. Loss of vitality of the nerves causes the sight to become dimmed and it also weakens the elastic fibre in the muscles throughout the entire body, allowing it to twist out of shape at many different points. This interferes with the circulation, causing the body to lose much of its motor power.

The physical imbalance that results from weakness of the nervous system can cause many different ailments although these can be avoided and are not irreversible. If the hormonal output is unbalanced, depression, emotional upsets and even suicide attempts can occur, even though to an outsider there is no apparent reason. Some of the mood swings are caused by an unexplained bio-chemical change in the brain, while others just seem to come over us.

Depression is experienced in different ways and with varying severity. The symptoms can include sadness, tiredness, disinterest, lack of concentration, loss of appetite or over-eating, insomnia or inability to get out of bed in the morning, and bouts of crying. At times it can become a serious form of anxiety and a fear for the future which can be quite debilitating. Certainly at mid-life it is not unusual to experience depressive periods, because of the fluctuation in hormone levels. A direct hormone connection can be a tremendous influence even during the pre-menopausal years. But I must emphasise that willpower, understanding and strength are important when one really feels desperate. Although this experience is more common in mid-life than at other times, let us not forget that such feelings hit all of us at some time or another during our life. Always identify the real problem and learn to relax. Do not make any major decisions while going through such a period, but take your time. There are many ways of diverting one's thoughts in order to gain time. So often, professional responsibilities or one's role in the family can stand in the way of overcoming depression. We may lack strength or feel useless and no longer required, especially if the family has grown up and gone their separate ways. If depression is menopause-related, the severity of the symptoms can vary because of a woman's individual biochemistry. To become calmer and attain a more peaceful state of mind, steps can be taken by way of diet, exercise, relaxation, or by supplementing with vitamins, minerals and trace elements. All these factors can influence us positively to overcome depressive bouts more quickly or even to avoid their occurrence all together.

Depression has been the subject of a considerable number of research projects. It has been discovered that women who have undergone a hysterectomy are more subject to clinical depression, especially those who have lost the uterus at a relatively early age. Marital problems after a hysterectomy can be the first sign of these depressive feelings and, more often still, diminished sexual desire. This of course can be overcome with the help of medical counselling. Depression, anxiety or mood changes can be helped by a positive attitude with a view to balancing the brain. This can be achieved by diet or herbal remedies, but the best cure of all is if the person is made to understand that she is loved. However, the conclusion of several studies is that it is not uncommon for women with menopausal depression to suffer mood swings, varying between depression and a more relaxed, cheerful and more self-contained stage. It just shows the importance of balance and that strong medication is rarely required. More often than not, with counselling or a partner's interest or love, the situation can be reversed. Some simple exercises can also be very beneficial and this is the reason why I always suggest making some time available for a healthy and relaxing pastime. There is no need for strenuous exercise, but some gentle jogging, cycling or swimming will benefit the condition, as insomnia is often another side-effect. The best advice I can give anyone is not to get frustrated and not to be too proud to ask for help. There is no shame attached to this condition and good and timely advice can prevent a lot of further problems. Try and cultivate a sense of humour and always remember that many more muscles are needed for a frown than there are for a smile.

There are of course various kinds of depression. The two main kinds are endogenous and exogenous depression. The first results from hormonal and biochemical changes in the body while the latter is influenced by outside factors. Sometimes it is difficult to differentiate between stress, anxiety and depression because in all of these problems the emotions play a major part. There is, however, no doubt that a poor diet and an imbalance of nutrients, vitamins, minerals, trace elements and enzymes play a major role in depressive illness. I often find that the remedy valerian is of great help for such conditions. When we look into history at the fashions in medicine it is quite amazing that way back in early civilisation, Hippocrates – the father of medicine – advocated valerian for women who were nervous or impatient. Today the potential of this herb has found renewed recognition and it is another herb with a message: it has many pointers that suggest it would serve us well in the treatment of the nervous system, and certainly for depression it is of great help. Jayvee, a remedy made by Nature's Best, contains natural extracts of valerian, *Crataegus* (hawthorn), *Humulus lupulus* (hops), *Viscum album* (mistletoe), passiflora and zinc. As an extra nerve tonic I confidently advise patients to use Dr Vogel's *Avena sativa*, which is an extract of oats, primarily designed for the strengthening of nerves, insomnia and irritability. It relaxes and promotes a healthier nervous system.

It is often said that depression only exists in the mind. If we can discover which fuse malfunctions or has blown, we will soon regain the balance. The nervous system works like a railway: if the train is on the rails, every fuse relating to the signals must be in the right place before the train can safely be driven. The hormone system is like the railway: everything works well, every hormone reaches its destination, when the fuses in the signal box are wired to the correct connections. Let's be positive and hope that we have the strength and the will when it is necessary. I am sure that we'll overcome our problems and eventually will be much richer and happier for having come through this phase.

Chapter 7

Forgetfulness and Insomnia

IT IS SURPRISING how much medical knowledge can be gleaned from old writings and documents. Manuscripts dating from times when all medicine was based on nature, some of them originating from the ancient celtic druids, reveal much that is relevant to medicine today. Unfortunately many of the old ways have been forgotten or overtaken by chemical-based medication.

Two frequently mentioned symptoms of the menopause are forgetfulness and insomnia. We have learnt of some old and tried natural remedies which can be of help for these specific complaints. I have already said that nature will often give us a clue as to the remedial properties of plants, but we are not always able to interpret these clues. For example, take a look at a leaf of the *Ginkgo biloba* tree. According to messages contained in medieval poetry, the *Ginkgo biloba* tree was worshipped by the Japanese and referred to as the 'Japanese temple tree'. If we place a leaf of this tree under the microscope and study its texture, we see that it resembles our brain. Moreover, if you take a leaf and chew it the brain will react immediately. This tree was clearly given to mankind as a remedy to assist in the function of the brain. No wonder that the Japanese considered it a holy tree. Not so long ago, on a visit to Switzerland, Dr Vogel took me to his first house where he proudly pointed to a *Ginkgo biloba* tree in his garden. He had it brought over to Switzerland many years ago. It had grown well and he was fascinated by it and had studied its characteristics for a long time. Eventually he decided to use this tree as the basis for a remedy Ginkgoforce, better know as Geriaforce. The fresh extract obtained by Dr Vogel has proved to be of great help for the memory and Geriaforce is now widely prescribed for forgetfulness.

The other day I was reading some German poetry and quite by accident I came across a poem written in 1815 by Goethe. He sent it to his assistant, accompanied by two leaves of the *Ginkgo biloba* tree:

> The leaf of this oriental tree, entrusted to my garden, has a secret of
>   which insiders only are aware.
> Selected and apparently divided, yet known as a single entity.

It proves that Goethe knew about the *Ginkgo biloba* tree, and in his poetry he intended to pass on his knowledge of its remedial properties. This tree contains ingredients which make it one of the finest remedies for people who become forgetful. The *Ginkgo biloba* is the world's oldest living tree species. Its lineage stretches back many centuries and, although it originated in China, it successfully grows to a ripe old age in the many other parts of the world to which it has been transplanted.

Modern scientific analysis revealed that the reason *Ginkgo biloba* trees have survived for so long may be that their leaves are packed with highly active chemicals that give the tree unusual resistance to parasites, infections and pollution. The leaves of the *Ginkgo biloba* tree are traditionally harvested in the autumn, just as the colour changes, because this is exactly the time when they contain the highest possible concentrations of active bioflavenoids. *Ginkgo* bioflavenoids are now thought to be the most potent of all, and it has been suggested that they have the ability to assist in maintaining the circulation of blood to the brain. The high biological activity of the *Ginkgo*'s ingredients also make the extract a powerful free radical scavenger which means that it has the ability to absorb and neutralise toxic chemicals within the body.

Ginseng is another well-known energy-giving remedy for forgetfulness. This is the world's best-known and most highly researched adaptogen, a substance that assists the body to adjust to unusual situations. In the Far East ginseng has been used for thousands of years, but it is only recently that it has become popular in the West. Ginseng forms the basis of another well-known Bioforce product, Ginsavena. This is a fresh herbal preparation, which is especially useful for lack of concentration, and, as the name indicates, its main ingredient is ginseng, combined with *Avena sativa*. An even stronger remedy, such as Ginsavita (also from the Bioforce range) will promote convalescence as well as physical and mental productivity, and contains the same basic ingredients, but of a higher potency. These remedies, prescribed in combination with Nature's Best's Imuno-Strength, will be of great help in overcoming forgetfulness.

Another widely experienced symptom of the menopause is sleeplessness or insomnia. This is often a direct result of night sweats, but there can also be other reasons. All too often any change in life's rhythm, or any inconvenience, is blamed on the menopause, which is not always justified. There are different types of sleep and in fact the definition of sleep is really different levels of unconsciousness. At times we sleep lightly, but there are also times when we sink into a really deep sleep. Our sleeping pattern often changes as we get older. Mostly our body requires less sleep as we get older and this is sometimes confusing.

I believe in the theory that the health of the lymphatic system is essential to our general health, because of its cleansing and purification function. Our lymph glands are constantly exposed to invaders and toxicity necessitates internal cleansing. It is important to recognise that this cleansing or purification mostly takes place during sleep and that is why it is so important that the body is allowed a healthy measure, i.e. on average approximately seven or eight hours sleep a night. Of course the amount of sleep required varies depending on the individual. I actually need more sleep than most people. I know that this is the time when my energy is replenished and I do not function in optimal form unless I have seven hours sleep. Some people may need no more than four hours; however, others cannot face the day unless they have had ten hours of sleep. These requirements vary from person to person and also depend upon how well we relax while asleep.

The way we prepare ourselves for the night is important and it surprises me to learn that some people use stimulants in the misguided belief that this will wear them out and enable them to have an unbroken sleep. This is not the way it works. Unfortunately, during the menopause women frequently experience sleeping problems and in desperation they will sometimes seek solace in sleeping tablets. I am not in favour of this because, although it may ensure a reasonable night's rest, there is a possibility of addiction; what the body really needs is to find its own rhythm. There are many natural substitutes which are not addictive or habit-forming. Try taking some light exercise or a warm bath in the evening, a herbal drink, or perhaps do some Hara breathing exercises.

I hear more and more often that people with sleeping problems have become television addicts. Many families nowadays appear to have a television in their bedroom and indeed I am even more disturbed at how common this is among youngsters. A whole new generation is growing up with the idea that this is perfectly normal. Often people who are afraid of not being able to drop off to sleep switch on the television hoping for some distraction and instead they get engrossed in an exciting programme, and then are surprised if they are unable to relax when they eventually shut their eyes or retire to bed. Under these circumstances problems with hot flushes and spontaneous perspiration become more common. Patients often remark that they stay up later because of interesting television programmes, drinking coffee and nibbling goodies until it is time to retire. The invention of television has been the cause of major changes in our way of life; this will be corroborated by market researchers. Our eating habits have changed so considerably that furniture manufacturers have designed tables especially for the purpose of enabling us to eat our meals while, at the same time, watching television. Food manufacturers happily advertise specific television meals and snacks. The variety of savoury snacks and nuts has grown beyond recognition as it is relaxing to sit and munch a little while watching the screen. Let me warn you that trying to get to sleep on a full stomach is not a good idea. The last meal of the day should be at least four hours before going to bed. Instead of sitting down to watch television, a short walk or some deep breathing exercises will improve the digestion and ensure a good night's sleep.

It is common to hear the menopause blamed for anything and everything. Take care to eliminate possible factors that can cause irritating problems which are not directly relevant to the menopause, and follow Dr Vogel's advice by using Dormeasan. This is not an addictive remedy but a mixture of herbs, some of which I have mentioned already:

Melissa officinalis (balm)	40%
Avena sativa (oats)	38%
Passiflora incarnata (passion flower)	10%
Humulus lupulus (hops)	9%
Valeriana officinalis (valerian)	2%
Lupulinum (hop grains)	1%

Dormeasan has a calming effect on people who have a tendency to over-excitement, restlessness and mental exertion. The difficulty arises when one becomes used to not sleeping or having a frequently interrupted sleeping pattern. In such cases I have found that acupuncture is of great help in breaking a long-standing habit. It is unwise to endanger the body's ability to respond in a natural way. A generally reliable method is reading for 15 or 20 minutes before going to sleep, or a gentle massage. In my book *Body Energy* I have described several massage methods that will aid relaxation and counteract insomnia. I have already pointed out that a warm bath is relaxing, and in my book *Water – Healer or Poison* many water treatments are listed, among them many methods developed by Father Kneipp. Fresh vegetable juices are also conducive to relaxation, such as carrot juice, celery juice or salad juice. Hot drinks to aid relaxation include lemon balm and tea or, if you are a coffee drinker, try Dr Vogel's Bambu coffee, which has a very pleasant taste and yet is not a stimulant. I have also seen positive results when people take Oil of Evening Primrose. It is advisable to take three 500mg capsules during the evening. Indeed, the naturopathic practitioner has much to offer, without incurring the risk of side-effects for the long-term use of drugs. Manipulative treatment can also be helpful for insomnia. I have helped many insomniacs with acupuncture or manipulative treatment.

Sometimes it may be helpful to follow an all-fruit diet for a few days, and even a grape diet can be beneficial. Indeed, a low-stress diet is of great help for sleeplessness. Sometimes insomnia can be the result of a physical condition: if that is the case, immediate action must be taken. It is imperative that the active side of the nervous system is given the chance to rest during the night. The breathing, digestion and absorption processes, and some of the fluid circulation are taken care of by the vagus nerve – the tenth cranial nerve. With this knowledge we can understand why cranial osteopathy is often useful. This is still a little-known or understood therapy, but is of great comprehensive holistic therapeutic value. By using these methods it is possible to effectively treat almost any condition. Personally I often practise it for emotional disturbances, and it is also effective for promoting general health and energy, balancing and integrating the whole person. The benefit of cranial osteopathy is that it is extremely gentle, but nevertheless should only ever be practised by a fully qualified practitioner. It works on a profound level, influencing the central nervous system and penetrating deeply. I have certainly seen many people with insomnia problems who have benefited from this gentle manipulation. Make sure that your bed is comfortable, neither too hard, nor too soft. If suffering from back or neck problems, which can be a hidden cause of sleeplessness, do some sensible exercise. Good sleep is essential if you want to have plenty of energy to cope with the requirements of a demanding job during the day.

Chapter 8

Post-Menopausal Conditions

IN THE *Pharmaceutical Journal* of 22 September 1990 Professor
Robinson explained that after the menopause the vaginal tissue,
epithelium, undergoes tremendous thinning – from around 50 to four
cell layers thick. A lack of fluid secretion means the tissue becomes
very dry and sore. In addition, and related to the lack of oestrogen,
the vaginal pH changes from acidic to almost neutral. Because of this,
the normal colonisation of lactobacillus is reduced and there is often
an overgrowth of other organisms, leading to bacterial and fungal
infection. Bioadhesive polymer has been found to produce a 20 per
cent increase in the flow of blood into vaginal tissue and this results in
a return of the tissue to its hydrated state. Being acidic, it also allows a
return to acidic pH, which suggests that bladder and vaginal
infections should be reduced.

Women in the early stages of the menopause often wonder what
life will be like after the menopause, despite the obvious attraction
that there need be no further fear of pregnancy and the added benefit
of no longer having to rely upon contraceptive methods. Yet, there is

a major concern: will it be possible to enjoy life as much as before the menopause? Actually, life has a lot to offer after the menopause, although some considerations may have to be remembered. I often quote a colleague of mine, Paavo Aerola, for whom I have a high regard. We have often lectured together and his following statement has always impressed me because of its insight: 'The menopause is a divinely designed phase in a woman's life, with the purpose of liberating her from her duties as procreator with God and giving her time for self-improvement, for the perfection of the human and divine characteristics and her spiritual growth.' This is how I also see it. After the menopause there is something to work for, both for the satisfaction of oneself and others.

The most common questions relating to the post-menopausal stage are about vaginal dryness. Moisture is essential for vaginal comfort and health. Unless moisture is present, all sorts of problems can occur, including itching and irritation, a feeling of pressure inside the vagina, and even pain during intercourse. It is widely believed that more than three million women in the UK regularly experience problems with vaginal dryness and most women will suffer from it at some time in their lives. Although it is by no means considered a serious medical condition, no woman wants to live with vaginal dryness. The most common symptoms are not restricted to menopausal women; they can also occur in breast-feeding women and women using certain contraceptive techniques. However it is during the menopause that they are most common: while the incidence of vaginal dryness is thought to be less than ten per cent at the age of 20, this figure rises sharply to approximately 35 per cent among women at the age of 50. Statistics indicate that 26 per cent of pre-menopausal women experience dryness sufficient to interfere with sexual intercourse and this rises to 45 per cent in pre-menopausal and post-menopausal women. Although there are quite a few products on the market for just this complaint, I have suggested that my patients try out some different lubricants and I must say that I have been amazed with the feedback on a product that has only recently appeared on the market. A double-blind evaluation of the moisturising gel Replens suggested effective action as a lubricating jelly in the treatment of vaginal dryness for pre-menopausal and post-menopausal women. The participants were separated into two groups and 80 per cent of the women who used Replens were satisfied. The efficacy response was determined by comparing the improvement within and between the two groups with regard to:

a) Vaginal cytology (i.e. the condition of the cells)
b) Vaginal pH
c) Duration of adherence to vaginal vault
d) Improvement in vaginal dryness index
e) Coverage of vaginal wall (comparison of photos)
f) Evaluation of the patients' diaries

Most people rate the gel from excellent to very good, and in comparison with other products it proved very satisfactory. A further benefit is that it is easy to use. In conclusion Replens was considered a superior product to other jellies that are available. In a six-month follow-up report in a multi-centre trial the results were more than satisfactory. Elasticity, a variable that did not show significant change in earlier short-term studies, was graded higher in the eventual report. This was significant as it may imply that long-term use of Replens may result in additional benefits. At six months, pH with Replens was statistically significantly lower than with competitive products. In 77 per cent of the participants the moisturiser took care of the vaginal dryness, while 15 per cent used another product, such as contraceptive foam. Sixty-three per cent of the women did not need additional lubrication at the time of sexual intercourse, while 30 per cent used an external lubricant. Forty-six per cent of the patients experienced discharge from the vagina one day after use, 37 per cent on the night of use, while 13 per cent did not experience leakage at all. Thirty-eight per cent experienced leakage that necessitated wearing a pantyliner while in 62 per cent this was not necessary.

Statistically significant improvements were observed in sexual arousal, lubrication, absence of pain during intercourse, orgasm and vaginal penetration. Among the partners of the women who took part in the trial, no significant effects were noted in observations of the following: lack of sexual interest, difficulty obtaining or maintaining erections, ejaculating too quickly, ejaculating too slowly or not at all, or experiencing pain during sex.

A study was also made of changes in vaginal blood flow patterns in post-menopausal women using Replens and a comparison was made between the changes occurring in women using Replens and women undergoing hormone replacement therapy. It was found that Replens induced an increase of vaginal blood flow comparable to that seen with hormone replacement therapy. This percentage change is similar to that seen in studies of vulva blood flow in post-menopausal women.

Replens owes its development to an emerging science known as bioadhesive technology. Unlike messy and old-fashioned lubricating jellies, this product actually restores moisture to the vaginal surface and continues moisturising and providing comfort throughout the day and night, so there is no need to use a lubricant just before intercourse. The key ingredient in Replens is polycarbophil. This has the ability to hold large amounts of moisture which it then passes to the vaginal tissues and, because polycarbophil adheres, the effect is longer lasting. Feedback from users suggests that Replens is able to replenish vaginal moisture for up to three days.

Replens is not a drug, but a completely natural way to replenish vaginal moisture. Clinical tests have shown that it is well tolerated and can be used with complete confidence for the long-term relief of vaginal dryness. It will improve a woman's comfort and confidence even more if she chooses to use Replens three times a week on a regular basis. I mention confidence because many patients have told me that without vaginal moisture, they regard sexual intercourse as a painful and embarrassing experience. Therefore regular use of Replens can restore confidence and once again make sexual relationships with one's partner a fulfilling experience for both. The product comes in easy-to-use, pre-filled disposable applicators. When used as directed, three times a week at bedtime, Replens is certain to end vaginal dryness every minute of every day.

It is quite enlightening to read some of the background statistics on the menopause. I have already mentioned that an estimated three million British women suffer from vaginal dryness, approximately a third of the presumed ten million women in the menopausal age group. Approximately 1,100 gynaecologists each see on average 400 menopausal women in a year, while annually 331,000 visits to general practitioners are made by menopausal women.

Sometimes I advise the use of vitamin E oil to lubricate the vagina and heal the dry tissues, especially if there have been some eruptions. Apply and gently massage the oil into the inner sides of the vagina. Among the available creams for this purpose, the one that seems to be most beneficial, according to feedback from my patients, is the Seven Herb Cream from Dr Vogel.

Another condition experienced by some women after the menopause is extreme itching, known as *pruritus vulvae*, which is very distressing and extremely embarrassing. This condition needs immediate treatment and should be investigated by a doctor or gynaecologist. However, whatever you do, don't let this put you off from a normal sexual relationship.

It is very important that a woman does not view her condition after the menopause in a negative light. Approach it positively and remember that sometimes it helps to concentrate on a new hobby, for example music. In some of the underdeveloped countries I have visited, I have seen women of 100 years and over, who were still able to use sound vibrations for their healing effects. Vibrations are important. Sir Arthur Eddington stated: 'When an electron vibrates, the universe shakes.' If this river of life is allowed to work its way through our body, harmonically and rhythmically, it will positively affect the energy fields in our body. The influence of positive vibrations should be appreciated for their remedial value.

I remember a particular lady who was so obsessed by her post-menopausal condition that even after the age of 60 she still felt the same as she did during the menopause. I informed her of the value of positive thinking and the power of vibration, and I also enquired if she had ever considered taking up singing or music, or in fact doing anything at all to encourage positive vibration. She accepted my advice after I explained the importance of the endocrine system, not only during the pre-menopausal and post-menopausal stages, but during the whole of our lives. I explained about the vibratory nature of our make-up, the vibrant expressions of a harmonious life, and also the beauty of life. I illustrated this theory by explaining that the seven endocrine glands are receptive to the seven colours in the solar spectrum, the seven layers of light receptors in the retina and the seven basic steps of a musical scale, which can be so important for harmony in our lives.

The body is really quite a wonderful invention. Just imagine that there are millions of very tiny receptors in the eye for perceiving and translating light waves into electrical impulses. These impulses stimulate the endocrine glands. The light waves correlate with the seven glands and each of these glands gives energy. In his wonderful book *Behold Man*, Lennart Nilsson shows some photographs of very tiny crystals: cortisone crystals contain pink spirals, insulin sparkles yellow and blue, while adrenalin darts across the camera lens in streaks of fiery orange, and oestrogen appears white with pink and blue spines, emerging spherically and invisibly contrasted by light red testosterone crystals that reflect the entire spectrum. Progesterone is a diamond-shaped white, green, blue and pink crystal with a white light in the centre. It's wonderful to see the life in those little crystals, life in general, but especially the life of a woman who indeed has a lot more to put up with than a man. Considering the physical discomforts in the life of a woman, we can indeed understand the saying that it's a man's world. And yet, being a woman has so many benefits and advantages. The specific stages in the life of a woman enable her to fulfil a variety of roles, e.g. wife, mother and a man's best friend. Where would man be without her?

If we look at it from this angle isn't life just wonderful? Isn't it great that together we can face the obstacles put in the way, which eventually serve to make us into stronger and better people?

Chapter 9

Hormone Replacement Therapy

WHEN I HAVE a surgery in my London clinic I always travel by underground from the airport, and sitting on the train recently I overheard a conversation between two women which was relevant to the subject of this chapter. I admit that it is bad manners to listen in to other people's conversations, but sometimes you just can't help it. I found the conversation interesting because they were discussing a subject which I am so often asked to deal with in my surgery, namely the menopause. These two ladies compared notes on their individual experiences and I heard one lady claim that prior to the menopause she often felt dizzy and was astonished at the lapses in her concentration. She also complained about the change in the quality of her hair and fingernails. Although still audible to me, she lowered her voice and informed her friend that she no longer had any appetite for sex and was plagued by cystitis. She had heard mixed reports about HRT and eventually decided to find out for herself. She had talked herself into setting up an appointment with her doctor, but was told that in her condition it was probably not advisable because of a history of cancer in her family. However, she had decided to ignore the doctor's advice. After a few months she claimed that she felt quite a bit better and a year later she felt absolutely wonderful.

The other lady had listened attentively and it wasn't until now that she volunteered that she too had considered HRT but was scared of possible side-effects. Therefore, as long as no assurances could be given, she had decided that she was better off suffering the hot flushes and trying to get through the menopause in the natural way, rather than facing the increased risk of developing breast cancer. To me she made a lot of sense and I was pleased to hear that she claimed her philosophy in life to be that where possible she would choose natural options in favour of chemical remedies. At this point, I'm sorry to say, the train stopped and both ladies left the compartment.

I continued my journey and mulled over the ladies' conversation even though I had heard nothing new. I often hear the first lady's point of view explained in my own surgery. There is no doubt that HRT can bring relief from menopausal symptoms. However, let's bear in mind that the feedback from many HRT users may well be slightly exaggerated and some women, if they are honest with themselves, will agree to this.

The subject of HRT often crops up in public lectures and is of great concern to women. In general it seems that the attitude of many 50-year-old women is that they have little to lose and much to gain. So why should they be stopped by some old fuddy-duddies in the medical profession? They believe that their skin and their sex life improve; there are no more hot flushes, and an added benefit is that it seems to protect against osteoporosis as well.

Unfortunately on several occasions I have seen patients who were possible victims of HRT and as a naturopathic practitioner this has been enough to make me be extremely wary of condoning HRT treatment. In naturopathy we practise the philosophy of effecting only minimal changes in the body, especially if they could result in apparently unconnected problems later. Who can honestly claim that HRT is without any long-term and still unknown side-effects, even for future generations?

There are too many unanswered questions. Does one prescribe HRT treatment for diabetics or for women with fibroid problems or a degenerative disease? Is HRT a body-builder or a body-breaker and will it benefit the immune system? As long as there is any doubt about the eventual outcome I must agree with a cautious approach. Certainly if the person concerned feels that she can no longer cope and the natural approach does not appear to be effective, it may have to be reconsidered. There is no doubt that HRT will bring relief for some symptoms, yet why not leave this method until alternative methods have been given a fair chance? Many women who have started HRT treatment expecting to feel and look years younger, have been extremely disappointed. HRT cannot regain women their youth.

The major question is whether or not HRT is indeed without side-effects. Basically, HRT is a method of replacing female oestrogen hormones which are thought to be deficient in menopausal women. This shortage may be responsible for symptoms such as night sweats, hot flushes, depression and osteoporosis. At this stage in life oestrogen and progesterone are produced in smaller quantitites or not at all. Therefore progesterone is also supplemented, especially for women who have had a hysterectomy. Sometimes a combination of these two hormones is prescribed. HRT may provide relief for the main symptoms and is thought to provide protection against the onset of osteoporosis, which affects males and females beyond a certain age. It must be remembered that not all women feel well on HRT and I have seen side-effects that were more bothersome than the initial symptoms. Some of the women I have seen have voluntarily discontinued the treatment. HRT will not stop the clock of nature, nor will it provide us with everlasting youth. There are other ways of keeping young and I have several friends who have reached the grand age of 100 and still have an active mind. The last thing they would consider is taking oestrogen and progesterone, which after all are artificial forms of originally natural supplements produced by the body.

Contradictory results of studies make us wary. There have been claims of increased risk of breast cancer or degenerative diseases. It is not absolutely certain that this treatment is safe beyond doubt and it is an individual's right to decide whether to use HRT or natural means. Let me stress, however, that if a decision has been made to use HRT, follow your doctor's advice and remain under his supervision. Although all women in the menopausal age group should have regular medical checks, it is absolutely essential for HRT users.

Let me stress that the liver is the regulator of our health. This organ may be compared to an efficient laboratory with a lot of work to do. It is a very busy laboratory and oestrogen taken by mouth has to pass through the liver where the production of proteins is stimulated. This can be helpful, but can also cause indigestion or raised blood pressure. Substances new to the liver can cause problems and cases of skin irritation and itchiness are not uncommon. In an attempt to avoid the necessity of hormone replacement I can think of many natural methods that assist the body in adjusting to new situations; dietary change and relaxation exercises are obvious measures, but there are also quite a few supplementary combinations which have proved to be worthwhile.

Some of the Ladycare formulae have proved to be extremely helpful and in that respect I would like to quote some information extracted from a report that was published on some of their research projects. This report is entitled: *A Little Knowledge is a Dangerous Thing (Women and their Understanding of Medical Problems)* and its opening statement is self-explanatory:

The findings from our survey showed a discrepancy between the desire to take responsibility for one's own health and having the knowledge to do that effectively.

Given that the main health fears with respect to the menopause are cancer and osteoporosis, are women sufficiently aware of how these diseases can be prevented? It would seem not. They have superficial knowledge and are often concerned and confused by the treatment they receive from doctors as it has not been properly explained nor have all the available options been discussed.

Although the majority of the study participants had undergone cervical smear tests and breast checks, they also registered a desire for more information about these illnesses, how they may be detected and then treated. Of all the age bands, the 40–49-year-old women appear to be the best informed. Younger women (under 39) and many in the 50-plus bracket agreed that they needed more information on breast cancer, cervical cancer and heart disease.

This lack of specified knowledge can probably be attributed to the individual woman as well as the sources of information – if women don't ask the right questions, then they won't get the right answers. But there is also something of the ostrich syndrome – if I ignore this disease, it may just go away. The assumption is that 'not all women contract cancer, so it is unlikely that I will be one of the unlucky ones'. Unfortunately statistics show that one in twelve women will develop breast cancer and, as a result, some of those women will die unnecessarily. Early detection is important, as a cure is then more likely. Nowadays doctors, clinics and hospitals prompt women to attend for cervical smear test screening, but the same cannot be said about symptoms of the menopause and attendant ailments.

The women surveyed in our research were asked to list the symptoms of the menopause they knew about and nearly all of them were able to identify the more obvious, such as depression, irregular periods, hot flushes and night sweats. However, there was a demonstrable lack of understanding of how the body changes and the long term effects of hormonal imbalance and deficiency.

During the menopause women lose oestrogen which, in turn, causes great discomfort by making the vagina dry and inflamed; hormone deficiency also accelerates thinning of the bones – osteoporosis. Osteoporosis kills one in four women over 60, yet women's knowledge of how this condition can be prevented or treated is blatantly lacking. Seventy-four per cent and 66 per cent of the surveyed women know they are at risk from cervical and breast cancer (respectively), yet only 19 per cent recognised the dangers of osteoporosis. Seventy-two per cent agreed that they did not have enough information on this subject, including an alarming 63 per cent of women over 50 – the most susceptible group.

Hormone replacement therapy has been available for over 20 years to help alleviate the symptoms of the menopause, counteract osteoporosis and offer help against cystitis and heart disease. Although women were familiar with the term, many did not know enough about it, its benefits or possible side-effects. Again, the 40–49 age group were best informed, but nearly half of the 25–39 bracket knew nothing at all.

The Ladycare 2,000 survey report was especially interesting as a cross-section of lifestyles had been selected for participation.

The magazine *Women's Weekly* of 23 October 1990 featured an article written by Iona Smith, mentioning some of the historical facts of hormone replacement therapy. It stated that implants of the hormone oestrogen were first used in 1938, while oestrogen-containing pills were not available for use until 1974. The article continues by pointing out that there are still doubts about the treatment and that the main fear is that HRT can increase the risk of cancer of the womb. This is largely because in the early days of HRT oestrogen alone was given, which can lead to a build-up of the endometrium (the lining of the womb), increasing the risk of cancer. It is thought, however, that when a low dose of progesterone is added this chance is minimal. Unfortunately, in my clinics I have attended to a number of women who had been given HRT and contracted breast cancer. Of course, this does not prove conclusively that HRT is the cause of breast cancer, yet it does nothing to allay some of the existing suspicion.

I have also helped some severely depressed women and admit that HRT can also positively influence a patient. It is my experience, however, that HRT is not advisable for women with a nervous disposition, as the risk is too great. I would also advise women with thrombosis, fibroids, endometriosis, diabetes, and gall-bladder problems to be specially careful. At this stage in a woman's life the body changes very quickly and some of the things that we normally take for granted can change overnight.

The hypothalamus and the pituitary glands function as regulators, producing and releasing agents, prompting the pituitary gland to manufacture hormones of its own and stimulate further production elsewhere. The hypothalamus is responsive to physical and emotional influences, while the pituitary gland starts the menstrual cycle by producing a hormone called follicle stimulating hormone, abbreviated to FSH. The follicles ripen in the ovaries. These grow and secrete a second hormone called oestrogen. This hormonal product acts on the lining of the uterus, causing it to thicken and grow. It is the oestrogen hormone that makes the breast and the vagina sensitive and directs the ovaries and, indirectly, the fallopian tubes. Ovaries need to be looked after very well as they shrink and harden after the menopause. With dietary measures or natural remedies it is possible to help the ovaries in this process of maturing or ageing naturally.

Protection in this particular age group can reduce the risks of ovarian cysts or even cancer. Ovarian cancer is most common in women in their sixties. During the menopausal period it makes sense to be alert for abdominal discomfort, indigestion or absorption problems. The same applies to osteoporosis. There is no definite need to use HRT in order to protect the body from osteoporosis. I have already mentioned the remedy Urticalcin and in this context I must again emphasise its beneficial properties. Also some of the specific menopausal formulae can protect and safeguard future health. After the menopause bones seem to break more easily and this is often due to calcium loss. Check that any calcium supplement is easily absorbed, and as well as Urticalcin, I can also recommend the remedy called Boron Plus from Nature's Best. This is a recently developed supplement of trace minerals which are essential and subtle arbiters of our health.

Trace minerals are needed in smaller amounts than other minerals and some vitamins, yet in some cases they seem to play just as important a role. They are fundamentally important because they are integral parts of the two types of biochemicals that perform or influence major functions in the body and brain, namely enzymes, which act as catalysts that trigger all the complex reactions we call metabolism, and hormones, which are the chemical messengers that switch on and off those reactions.

Trace minerals are partially lost in food refining and processing. Research has shown that even prime agricultural soils are sometimes deficient in minerals such as zinc and selenium. With the use of modern fertilisers it is quite possible to grow healthy looking vegetables and grains which contain only low levels of these minerals that are vital for human well-being.

Boron is an ultra-trace mineral that seems to be disappearing from the food chain due to modern agricultural practices and techniques. Although it is not generally agreed that it is essential in the diet of man, recent research has indicated that boron may have a role in human metabolism whereas previously it had been pigeon-holed as of little interest. Now boron is attracting attention on two fronts. Firstly, some American research suggests that boron acts as a pathway for oestrogen, the natural hormone that helps lay down calcium and maintain healthy bones. It is also thought to assist in vitamin D metabolism and it appears to be involved with balancing levels of oestrogen and testosterone. Secondly, boron may act as a membrane catalyst in cells, releasing energy that can be used to regenerate cartilage and collagen, the connective tissues that are of prime importance for smooth-working joints. Fibres of collagen thread through bones and help to give them their incredible strength.

New Boron Plus has been formulated exclusively for Nature's Best by Derek Bryce-Smith, Professor of Organic Chemistry at Reading University, and co-author of *The Zinc Solution*. This remedy supplies key co-factors, calcium, magnesium and vitamins D and B_2 riboflavin.

I certainly believe that a menopausal woman ought to give these remedies a chance first, rather than using harsher methods. By so doing many women have been able to avoid progressing on to unnatural and chemical therapies, such as HRT.

A disconcerting article appeared in the *Daily Mail* of Friday 22 February 1991 under the title 'Crisis of Women in Misery', sub-titled 'Hormone clinics are swamped as family doctors refuse to help'. It reads as follows:

Health Service centres providing hormone replacement therapy face a crisis. They are being swamped because many doctors refuse to help, according to a recent survey.

Almost 40 per cent of women suffer from symptoms caused by the menopause for more than five years, before they seek help from a specialist clinic. At least one in three women trying to cope with symptoms ranging from hot flushes to depression finds her family doctor uninterested or unhelpful.

'The few menopause clinics which exist are vastly oversubscribed, with a potential deterioration in the level of care offered,' said consultant gynaecologist Mr John Studd, who led the survey.

Many attending the handful of specialist clinics available on the NHS have had to take the initiative themselves, according to the study done at Dulwich Hospital in south-east London, and published in the *Journal of the Royal Society of Medicine*.

Nearly half the women attending the clinic referred themselves, and of those sent by GPs half said it was at their suggestion rather than that of a doctor.

Over twenty per cent of 150 new patients surveyed at the Dulwich clinic had travelled more than 20 miles. Many patients had been suffering for years but had not sought help for some time because they thought the symptoms would eventually get better. But one in four did not know that help was available.

Only 13 per cent had safety fears about HRT that had put them off seeing a doctor sooner.

HRT replaces essential hormones no longer produced after the menopause when ovaries cease to function. It combats symptoms and protects against potentially life-threatening conditions like heart attacks and rapid bone loss.

There are currently 24 free NHS menopause clinics, of which 17 are based in teaching hospitals where research is carried out. The hospital clinics cannot answer the general problem, said Mr Studd. Most see so many patients they are fast approaching saturation point. Mr Studd wants more clinics in the community and more GPs to prescribe HRT without referring patients to hospital.

The final sentence of the article, stating that more clinics in the community should be founded so that women would not have to be referred to hospitals, causes concern. With all respect to doctors, I am worried, because some of the women I have attended to and who had received HRT had not been monitored at all. Never forget that prevention is better than cure, and to my mind the natural way must always be considered as the first option.

The excuse is often that times have changed and I agree that life for women in the twentieth century is demanding. Many women are very busy, because as well as bringing up children, they also have a professional career. HRT treatment may relieve menopausal symptoms more quickly, allowing women to continue with their busy lives. However, a recent survey suggests that 92 per cent of women questioned believe that they should accept responsibility for their own health, and that more women worry about breast cancer (33 per cent) and cervical cancer (30 per cent) than any other disease. Forty-nine per cent worry about being overweight at some stage in their life. One third of all women smoke and 87 per cent have used some form of contraception.

I was pleased to read that a large majority of the women questioned wonder how the final decades of their life will be spent.

This awareness is excellent as on average a third of a woman's life takes place after the menopause. It is the lack of understanding that drives women to search for immediate relief, available either in the form of a patch, an injection or by oral administration.

The other day I saw a lady in my practice and looking at her I immediately suspected that she was hypertensive. Before I checked her blood pressure she told me about feelings of pins and needles, in her words funny feelings around her lips, and constant headaches. She informed me that she took no medication, only HRT. She had mentioned her concern to her doctor who had assured her that all was well. However, hypertension is listed as a possible side-effect of HRT. This lady was ill advised not to try a different method. If the decision is made to take HRT careful medical checks are essential, when regular examination of the breasts and a smear test of the cervix should take place.

A blood test will show if the liver is functioning well. A thyroid test will soon show if the seven endocrine glands are in harmony. Any HRT patient should be part of a careful monitoring programme and every few months tests should be performed. As long as there is no conclusive data or scientific evidence that HRT is absolutely safe I will continue to advocate that it makes more sense to use natural means.

If patients feel that they have reached the end of the road, then they must make the final decision, but not before being aware of any possible adverse effects. Natural remedies include Urticalcin, Boron Plus, Gynovite, Dr Vogel's Herbal Woman's Formula, or Oil of Evening Primrose. The ultimate decision must be the patient's. It must be her decision, but only after she has been given all the facts, which will allow her to make an informed choice.

Chapter 10

Diet

IT STANDS TO REASON that as a woman's body changes, so do her dietary requirements. The two most widely experienced changes during and following the menopause are both diet-related, i.e. an increase in body weight and fluid retention. Some relatively minor dietary changes can easily compensate for the physiological changes. Yet the nutritional value of food intake should not be allowed to suffer.

Having said this, I must clarify that over-nutrition can be as big a problem as malnutrition. One major problem that often arises is that the over-nourished eat far beyond their digestive capacity in both quantity and quality. It is especially quality that we have to look for in order to keep the hormone system happy, which, in turn, will keep the mind and body in good health. The digestive system is very important and the sort of foods that affect the digestive system negatively should be avoided.

It is universally believed that fruit, vegetables, nuts, seeds and sprouts are best for the health. Especially during the menopause, it is advisable to eat more often and in smaller quantities. Have a piece of fruit or a light snack at regular intervals – every three hours or so. The golden rule is to avoid excess protein, especially protein that induces toxicity. Remember that animal protein burns like coal in the fire, leaving clinker, and a good carbohydrate burns like wood in the fire, leaving no more than ash. Animal protein leaves its evidence in the form of energy blockages, while carbohydrates burn up quickly and can easily be eliminated from the body. Dairy food intake should be reduced and in some cases even avoided, especially as nowadays milk is often blamed for heart and circulatory problems. I must repeat that the intake of animal protein can often cause unnecessary stress in the body. Under these circumstances it is always better to follow a low-stress diet or a slimming diet, an example of which is featured towards the end of this chapter. Remember that food such as ice-cream, sweets, cakes and biscuits, and unnecessary salt, sugar and heated fats have no place in any healthy diet. The simpler the diet, the better one's health will be.

On a visit to India I was instructed in some basic rules which I have recommended to my patients, where applicable. These rules have proved very successful and yet they are simple. The day is divided into time bands with corresponding recommended foods. The period from 04.00 hours to 12.00 hours is the elimination cycle, when fruit should be eaten. The next time band is from 08.00 hours to 16.00 hours, the assimilation cycle, when not much of any food should be eaten. From noon until 20.00 hours is the digestive cycle and fruits, vegetables, nuts, seeds etc. can be eaten, with the specific advice to eat as much as possible of one's food raw. As I have received an excellent feedback from my patients on this programme, I would suggest that menopausal women should bear it in mind. Grains and legumes are also best eaten raw, where possible.

The body is quite content with fruits and vegetables as it is nearly impossible to eat too much of them, as long as we eat them separately and allow some time for digestion in between. For example, melon and bananas are jealous fruits and should always be eaten separately. Balancing foods, or food combining, holds the secret for feeling good and enjoying energy and good health. Good health is within everyone's reach; it only requires a little extra thought and some planning and insight. Its prerequisites are dietary sense and interest, pure drinking water, a clean environment and some physical exercise and activity.

From the point of view of osteoporosis, the diet should contain a sufficient intake of calcium, iron and other necessary minerals. The level of sugar in the blood must not exceed its advised limits. Automatic regulating processes are necessary to keep the blood sugar level balanced. An imbalanced sugar level can result in diabetes. With healthy people, when the sugar level rises to its upper limits, the mechanism ensures that the extra sugar is diverted to the urine, so that the blood sugar level is maintained below the limit. Similarly, if the blood sugar level drops to the lower limit, the balancing process comes into operation and, with a spurt of adrenalin, sugar is released from tissue cells and passed into the bloodstream. The blood sugar level is dependent upon our daily carbohydrate intake. Eating sugar will cause a very rapid rise, while starches work a little slower. Hence my advice to PMS and menopausal patients is to eat small portions of starchy food, potatoes or wholemeal products. Remember the rule to eat little and often. If you feel awkward because it isolates you from the rest of the family, consider that this rule may work just as well for the whole family. By eating less and more often many cases of hiatus hernia have been avoided. The fear of putting on weight can be eliminated, because digestive aids will be more helpful for smaller meals. As far as the weight problem is concerned, always remember that the effectiveness of any weight control is related to the degree of reduction in daily food intake. By that, I mean that by eating more often, one usually eats less. Make sure that the foods you eat are sufficiently rich in calcium, as it is important that the calcium levels are kept high in order to avoid osteoporosis. Calcium-rich foods include yoghurt, cottage cheese, cabbage, molasses, broccoli, tofu and tortillas. If you are in doubt about your calcium intake, please consider supplementing with Urticalcin. It is ironic, but great meat eaters have more problems with osteoporosis than vegetarians. Also remember that salt (sodium chloride) is detrimental to the health. Caffeine accelerates the loss of calcium from the body, and so the intake of drinks such as tea, coffee and colas should be carefully regulated, especially by menopausal women.

Let me also point out that because of the physiological changes in the body at this stage of a woman's life, unexpected allergic reactions may occur. Allergies are an intricate subject and must never be ignored. If you would like to know more about them I suggest that you read my book *Viruses, Allergies and the Immune System* which contains much general and specific information on this subject. Nutritional needs and susceptibility to allergic reactions vary with the individual, so expert advice may be useful. It is quite alarming to see how certain sensitive or allergenic foods can unbalance a menopausal woman's hormonal management system. Particular dietary care and awareness at this stage can easily avoid the need for medical treatment later.

Allow me to remind you of the dangers of the three Ss, i.e. salt, sugar and stress. Also I would ask you to avoid the use of artificial sweeteners, as I have seen too many problems where artificial sweeteners caused allergic reactions, eventually leading to other problems.

Although you may think this advice is complicated, never forget the invaluable benefits that can be gained from a healthy diet. One does not require an outstandingly clever mind to know whether a specific nutrient is good or bad for you. Once a person is used to a different dietary regime the slight effort it took to change one's habits will appear minimal.

Some time ago I was shocked to see a pitiful lady shown into my surgery. I soon learnt that during the early stages of the menopause she had taken to the bottle and now it was obvious that she was dependent on alcohol. She was by no means the first example I had seen, because it seems that women are much more prone to alcohol abuse during this stage in their lives. The love of her family had allowed her indulgence to develop into a severe problem before steps were taken to address it. No one had realised that this was not just a passing phase. Although the alcohol had temporarily eased her problems she had needed more and more to reach the stage of oblivion for which she searched. In this way she had damaged her brain cells and lost her sense of reality. She was no longer able to keep her house and look after the family the way she used to and the only pleasure she had to look forward to was the next drink. This lady from a caring family had changed rapidly and became a different person. The worst effect of alcohol is that it changes a person into a self-indulgent egotistical being. I spoke to the lady's husband and daughter and when I watched her leave I could only hope and pray that they would give her the positive support that she needed so badly. I had spoken harshly to her in the hope that she would listen and change her ways before it was too late.

A good diet can help to decrease one's dependence upon alcohol by replacing it with nourishing, wholesome food, uncontaminated with chemicals. Introduce rice and fish (especially herring, mackerel, sardines and white fish) into the diet. Fruit juices are also recommended, especially beetroot and carrot juice. Freshly grated beetroot and carrot, mixed with some apple juice and raisins makes a delightful and healthy side salad. There is not an awful lot of work required, and although it is often tempting to eat convenience foods, it is worthwhile to steer clear of junk foods which rob the system of good nutrition. Even if you are able to eat everything without gaining weight, don't be tempted to overeat. One's individual metabolic system decides how the body metabolises food.

Some people have made a lot of money out of designing and promoting fad diets. Be sensible about your dietary approach. There is no such thing as a universally effective slimming diet: any diet must be adjusted to suit individual lifestyles and metabolisms. I have composed a general diet for the purpose of weight reduction, taking into consideration health requirements, which the reader is advised to use as a foundation diet:

N.B. *The secret of success with this diet, as with all diets, is carefully weighing your food each time. All soups must be made using stock cubes and vegetables only. Cream soups may be made using part of your daily milk allowance.*

Daily allowances
Half pint of fresh milk, or one pint skimmed, or two cartons plain yoghurt
3oz wholemeal bread
4oz meat *or* 6oz fish *or* 4oz smoked fish *or* 5oz chicken

Weekly allowances
4oz butter or margarine *or* 8oz low-fat margarine
8oz cheese
Eggs (optional) up to seven maximum

Exchanges for 1oz bread

3oz potatoes
Two crispbread or crackers or water biscuits or plain biscuits
1oz breakfast cereal of any sort (except sugar coated)
   N.B. porridge uncooked weight
Two dessertspoons of cooked rice

Variety is the spice of life

Meats	4oz daily cooked any way, except fried
	Beef, corned beef, kidney, lamb, liver, mutton, tongue, tripe, sweetbreads, veal
or Fish	6oz daily, cooked any way, except fried – 4oz if smoked
	Cod, crab, haddock, halibut, hake, herring, kippers, lobster, ling, mackerel, mussels, oysters, pilchards, prawns, salmon, sardine, shrimps, trout, tuna
or Poultry/Game	5oz daily, cooked any way, except fried
	Chicken, turkey, rabbit, grouse, pheasant, venison
Eggs	One medium egg daily (optional) – not fried
Cheese	Caerphilly, Camembert, Cheddar, Cheshire, cottage cheese, Danish Blue, Edam, Gruyere, Leicester, Parmesan, Roquefort, Stilton, Wensleydale, smoked Austrian
	1oz daily of any of the above except cottage of which 4oz is allowed
Vegetables	No restrictions. Artichokes, asparagus, aubergines, bean-sprouts, Brussels sprouts, beetroot, broccoli, any type of cabbage, cauliflower, celery, carrots, cress, cucumber, courgettes, chicory, leeks, lettuce, marrow, mushrooms, onion, peppers, pimentoes, parsnip, parsley, French beans, runner beans, radish, swede, spring onions, spinach, pickles, tomatoes
In moderation	Peas, beans (butter, broad and haricot), baked beans (3.5oz), sweetcorn, avocado, chickpeas

Fruit	Three portions daily from:	
	apple – one average	peach – one average
	apricots – two fresh	pear – one average
	banana – one small	pineapple – one slice
	blackberries – 4oz	plums – two fresh
	cooking apple – one large	
		pomegranate – one small
	cherries – 4oz	prunes – six stewed
	dates – 1oz	raisins - 1oz
	damsons – ten	raspberries – 5oz
	gooseberries – ten	rhubarb – 5oz
	grapefruit – half	strawberries – 5oz
	grapes – 3oz	sultanas – 1oz
	melon – one average slice	
		tangerines – two
	orange – one average	
		juice – 4 fl.oz

Drinks	Tea (Russian tea, herb tea), coffee, Bovril, Oxo, Marmite, soda water, lemon juice, tomato juice, water, low calorie drinks, slimline drinks
Seasonings	salt, pepper, vinegar, mustard, lemon juice, herbs, spices, Worcester sauce

N.B. *Your daily allowance must be consumed within a period of 24 hours. Eat your weekly allowance within a week. You may eat as often as you like within your allowance. However, you must not eat less than three meals a day. If a food does not appear on this list do not eat it.*

The most important ingredient for any diet is willpower. Without it, you will never reach your goal. Whether it involves counting calories or taking food replacement drinks, the only way is to make up your mind that this is for your own good. The other day I made a lady very happy because I had advised her to halve all portions. When she came back to the clinic she claimed that she had never realised how easy it would be and she had lost a stone while hardly noticing that she was trying to lose weight. Sitting down and giving in does not burn up the calories. It is the quality of food and not the quantity that counts. After all, it is safe to say that we all need less food than we actually eat. Just bear in mind that one ounce of chocolate can be substituted for four tablespoons of carrots, without going over the limit. A cup of white sugar can be replaced by 1.3 cups of cane sugar or 1.5 cups of honey. You will not need this because it is too much. One cup of white flour is equivalent to seven-eights of a cup of wholewheat flour. When experimenting with substitutes you will always find that the healthier the food, the less you will need to eat. So please, make some dietary changes and the reward will be more than worth it.

Chapter 11

Essential Remedies

IT IS SOME 25 years since I first prescribed what was then a new remedy: Oil of Evening Primrose. At that time it was not yet available in Great Britain and I was ridiculed when I had it imported and prescribed in my clinic. The patients to whom I prescribed this remedy soon reported back gratefully. Today doctors can prescribe Oil of Evening Primrose for their patients on a National Health prescription and it is widely recognised for its outstanding properties. The seeds of the evening primrose are rich sources of essential fatty acids (EFAs) and in numerous cases the energy in those little seeds has restored the zest for life in menopausal women.

EFAs are as important a nutrient as vitamins and minerals. They cannot be made by the body and have to be supplied in our food. EFAs are required throughout the body and brain, since not only are they an integral component of cell membranes, but they are metabolised to form hormone-like substances known as prostaglandins, which control many metabolic pathways. One of the most important of these substances, prostaglandin El (PGE1), takes part in the control of the blood pressure, the stickiness of platelets in blood, the immune system and cholesterol production.

EFAs are polyunsaturated fatty acids. Before they can be metabolised to prostaglandins, they must be converted to even more unsaturated fatty acids such as gamma linolenic acid (GLA), a precursor of PGE1. Sometimes this conversion process is inefficient or blocked, e.g. by alcohol, and then a dietary source of GLA can be useful to bypass the blockage.

Human breast milk is one of the best known suppliers of GLA, and experts have tried to find a more convenient food source. The evening primrose seed is one of the richest natural sources of GLA. This plant's oil has now become the standard EFA and GLA supplement and is usually available in encapsulated form. Nature's Best Evening Primrose Oil is encapsulated with gelatin, glycerin and purified water. Incidentally, I would like to mention here that the brain contains high levels of polyunsaturated fatty acids. While the cells of our bodies are replaced continually, our brain cells die off at the rate of one per second.

As I have pointed out in the previous chapter, diet is a very important factor in the occurrence and severity of menstrual symptoms. Therefore I want to draw attention to the fact that fish is a rich source of essential oils. Although we know that Eskimos eat an extremely high-fat diet, they nevertheless seem to stay healthier than the average Westerner. Scientists think this may be because the fish oil consumed by Eskimos contains massive quantities of particularly protective fatty acids. One of these is Eicosapentaenoic acid (EPA), known to be a crucial component in the body's production of prostaglandins.

Cold-water oily fish, such as herring and mackerel, are rich in EPA, as well as other important fatty acids found in the Eskimo diet, such as Docosahexaenoic (DHA). EPA and DHA belong to a group of fatty acids known as Omega-3s. Like certain Omega-6 type fatty acids, which form prostaglandins, they play an indispensable part in cell membranes and help maintain normal cholesterol levels in the blood. Omega-3s, however, are thought to be much more effective than Omega-6s at keeping blood thin and circulation moving – even in extremely cold environments.

Our normal food supply does not always provide fatty acids of this type, and sometimes the body's own attempts to manufacture them from other dietary fatty acids are not very successful. These fatty acids are extremely susceptible to destruction and change according to oxygen supply and temperature exposure. Nature's Best High Potency EPA supplement is a rich marine lipid source of both EPA and DHA.

I am keen to use these oils because I have witnessed so many of the benefits. Let me immediately stipulate that in order to get the best results, Evening Primrose Oil must be used correctly. The word 'evening' in the name is significant, because the remedy should be used last thing at night, taking a minimum of three 500mg capsules. If taken last thing at night it also helps the lymphatic system in the elimination of toxins from the body. Nowadays the seeds of the evening primrose are cultivated in at least 15 countries. In common with other seed oils, Evening Primrose Oil is composed almost entirely of triglycerides. The fatty acid composition of Evening Primrose Oil is, with the important exception of GLA content, similar to that of other widely used vegetable oils, such as corn, safflower and sunflower oil. All the fatty acids in Evening Primrose Oil, other than GLA, are currently consumed in large amounts in some countries. Blackcurrant seed oil or borage oil are also high in GLA. However, the seeds of evening primrose have a hidden energy which exceeds any of the other seeds.

In the absence of EFAs in the diet, body functions become abnormal or impaired. This is because EFAs are required for the structural maintenance of all membranes in the body and because they are precursors of short-acting substances important in the regulation of prostaglandins.

To help women with their problems Nature's Best and Ladycare have both created several excellent remedies, e.g. Evening Primrose and Evening Primrose mixed with Borage. Ladycare has developed a remedy called Protection Formula, which is an especially effective supplement for women during or after the menopause.

The Ladycare 2000 survey report, commissioned on behalf of the manufacturers of a range of vitamin and dietary supplements (see chapter nine), aims to demonstrate the usefulness of supplements for women, analysing how their lives are conducted and recognising the pressures. The report is based on an extensive survey, canvassing the views of more than 650 women on issues affecting them. The women were asked a series of questions dealing with health, home life, family, career, and money, along with less tangible subjects such as their fears, aspirations and daydreams. The survey revealed that women would like to take more responsibility for their own lives and in particular for their health. However, although today's women want to take more positive action, they feel there is a lack of information to help them effectively. Whether through evolution or resolution, women find the resources to cope, the energy to care and the determination to make things happen.

As a result of this excellent survey, the Ladycare 2000 report also showed how a woman's body, and therefore her nutritional needs, change during her life cycle. It seems that most women are concerned about the absence of nutrients in their daily diet and with this in mind I thought it necessary to mention such excellent products as Optivite, Boron, and Health Insurance Plus. I am well aware that in the twentieth century women certainly do not have an easy life. Many women care for a family and run a home, as well as follow a career of their own, and fulfil social commitments, and by choosing to do so they are exposed to a great deal of pressure. When you add to all that the changing demands of the body in the different stages of a woman's life, it is not surprising that some women find it very difficult to cope. That is when some of these specific supplements can be so helpful.

When the production of oestrogen decreases, the menopause symptoms may continue for some time. Please don't see it as a weakness when help is needed to overcome or avoid the weariness of night sweats, insomnia, hot flushes, irritation, depression, and general nervous conditions. Some women see a hysterectomy as the solution, or a hormone preparation, but such drastic steps may not be necessary. Others are more sensible and opt for a vitamin E supplement, or zinc, or some homoeopathic or herbal remedies, which have no side-effects. Together with a healthy regime of fresh air, physical exercise (e.g. swimming or walking) and a good diet, a lot of unnecessary stress can be avoided or overcome.

There are numerous remedies for specific menopausal problems. The list is a long one, but it may be helpful to learn about a few of them. For example, sage will help prevent night sweats. Apis will take away the swelling of ankles and sensitive feet. Cimicifuga (*Actea racemosa*) is helpful for headaches, depression, feelings of gloom and hysterical fears. Graphite is useful for weight problems, especially abdominal ones. Hepar Sulph will take away irritability and anger, and also helps night sweats. Ignatia can help with mood swings, bereavement or grief. Lachesis is excellent for feelings of constriction and balancing the last menstruation problems. Lycopodium is helpful for anxieties, loss of self esteem, and for unspoken worries in connection with sexual performance. Natrium Mur often helps with weeping spells and bouts of impatience. Phosphorus is for headaches and prolonged, but light, periods. Pulsatilla deals with emotional sensitivity, lack of love and sympathy. Sepia is for irregular periods, irritability and distress. Staphisagria is for anger and resentment, guilt and sexual insecurity.

Dr Vogel has developed a formula which includes many of these components and has even added some others. This remedy is marketed as Formula MNP. This excellent homoeopathic remedy is of help for most menopausal problems. I have prescribed it for many of my female patients, nearly always with excellent results. If a course of Formula MNP is started early, as soon as problems arise, it will soon prove its effectiveness.

Twenty-three doctors took part in an interesting trial on this product and it was concluded that 75.8 per cent of women reported that it was an efficient remedy to end unwanted perspiration, which was noted as the biggest problem.

The term menopause literally means 'cessation of periods' and is derived from the Latin words 'mensis' (month) and 'pausa' (stop). However, over the years the meaning of the word has changed somewhat. It is important to understand the physiological changes which take place in a woman's body. During the reproductive period in a woman's life, the ovaries regulate the menstrual cycle by producing oestrogen and progesterone. It follows that when the production of these hormones ceases, essential supplements and remedies may be necessary. Although such physiological changes may result in mental and physical changes, one should remain positive and appreciate that help is available. The other day I treated a lady who was very depressed and she described it as being in a long black tunnel, unable to see the end. I quoted a passage from an article by Dr Vogel: 'Where there is shadow there is light, or there would be no shadow.'

The majority of women nowadays express a preference for homoeopathic or herbal treatment. Not long ago I received a grateful letter from a lady who thanked me for helping her successfully overcome the hot flushes and depression for which she had sought my advice. She had taken Optivite and Urticalcin and it had changed her life; so much so, that she now felt a new woman. Such feedback is helpful and encouraging for women who feel that they are suffering alone.

Chapter 12

Exercises

THERE ARE MANY ways in which a woman can help herself, probably more during the menopausal years than at any other time of her life. In the previous chapters I have concentrated on rules for healthy eating, and indicated the importance of avoiding stress, by not taking on more than is sensible, and by allowing time for the things you enjoy. In such a programme, exercise is very important. Exercise and diet are inseparable when striving to maintain good health, as both have a profound effect on the metabolic system. Correct and sensible exercise stimulates the metabolism. As the body's tolerance to certain foodstuffs depends to a large extent on our metabolic rate, exercise is a great influence. Active working people and children who keep busy have a higher tolerance to adverse dietary influences and allergies. It is a known fact that the less a patient exercises, the stricter he should be with his diet. Alternatively, if patients have difficulty in resisting danger foods, it is sensible to suggest that they take more exercise to burn up the bad food, increasing the metabolic rate to assimilate concentrated food and dispose of toxic food residues. Let us define what can be considered as correct exercise.

As an example I'll use the occurrence of a headache or a migraine. When the blood sugar level suddenly drops, it can trigger a migraine, and sudden physical exertion or physical or mental stress can easily result in a headache. A regular glucose trickle maintains a steady blood sugar level, and this can be aided by eating a healthy diet, including wholegrain foods. Regular and sensible exercise is required to curb allergic conditions. A good exercise schedule stimulates the flow of oxygen through the system, replenishing the oxygen in the muscle tissue. Incorrect exercise achieves the opposite, which is a depletion of the oxygen stored in the muscle tissue. Regular, sustained and comfortable exertion exercises the heart and leaves one feeling exhilarated, rather than exhausted and worn out.

Good forms of exercise are swimming, walking, cycling, or any sensible form of exercise which does not overtax the body. People often ask my opinion on aerobic exercises and of course there is a lot of benefit to be had from aerobics, but a sensible programme is important. Unfortunately I have had to treat many an aerobic enthusiast who has sought my help for osteopathic treatment. Excessive or unwise exercising can easily damage the back or muscular structure, and as an osteopath I must warn you that the goal of any exercising regime must be within the reach of one's physical abilities. By that I do not mean that if you cannot run a four-minute mile now, you never will be able to do so. By training or being trained sensibly, youngsters will be able to attain feats they may have considered impossible, but this is not what I am talking about. I am talking about the average person who does a bit of sport at the weekend or in the evening to stay in shape or maintain stamina. Do not drastically change your programme and delve into a new and exhausting pastime without guidance. Always use your common sense and by exercising regularly and sensibly, you may be able to move the goalposts.

Exercise in the way I advocate does not mean a lot of physical jerking. It means practising a daily routine of physical exercise, which helps the person mentally and physically. Exercise to achieve this must be introduced gradually and frequently practised. Imagine if by reading a book about the arts, one could become a singer. It isn't quite as simple as that. One needs to exercise and practise. Of course, all abilities or capabilities are gained by controlled practice, but a sign-post may put a person on the right road. For instance, look at the ease of the man who showed evidence of having enough vitality upon which to base magnetism, but who was often drained of energy by irrelevant emotions. He was nervous and fidgety and had no control over himself, or anyone else. He was told that he wasted a lot of his energy and he decided that enough was enough. A chance remark registered and he decided to act upon it. He managed to reduce his wasteful movements, his uneasiness, his nervous twitches, and was surprised to find that it required no more time or effort than was used by giving in to them. He resolved to master control, by refraining from all the nervous motions of hands, head, knees, feet and the body in general. He was determined to do something about it and, having conquered his fidgety movements, the drain on his energy and vitality eased. He found a new force of vitality and energy, without losing his magnetism, for he had learned how to use and channel this power.

This proves the tremendous value of storing up vitality. At first the man was like an engine that makes steam with all escapes open. Then, when he had learnt how to shut off the escapes, he was an engine of great power. The development of the most powerful form of personal magnetism must have been but a relatively easy step, because he had taken the trouble to learn about the simple process whereby it could be accomplished.

Thus we see that the correct method of exercising may be the start of habits that lead to the acquisition of such power. The practice requires a certain amount of time, but Rome wasn't built in a day. Time is required to train oneself to do things in a certain way, things that have to be done in any event.

In my book *Body Energy* I mentioned many ways of relieving stress by the use of one's own hands. With his permission I quote the following passage collated by Dr Leonard Allen, a very good friend of mine.

Hands ! ! !

The human hand is trained from infancy to express the thought or purpose of the mind which it controls.

The hand is the tool which the mind depends upon, when it wants to get anything done.

Thoughts of action naturally turn to the hand for their expression.

The hand is the first means of expression.

The baby uses the hand long before it learns to walk.

The savage who has but a few words in his vocabulary depends on the hand to express his thought.

The hand ministers; it carries aid.

The hand lifts the fallen, ministers to the sick. It is peculiarly the organ of expression of the good wishes of the kindly disposed.

When we are hurt, we instinctively place the hands upon the injured part.

When another suffers and we sympathise, we instinctively use the hand to soothe pain.

Clasped hands are the universal pledge of friendship and good will.

From the earliest dawn of civilisation, the hand has been used in the most sacred ceremonials.

The hand is the natural organ of expression, and its actions are mental symbols to which man had learned to make response through untold ages of experience and adaptation.

I would now like to instruct you on one of the best exercises I know, especially when feeling stressed during the menopause. This exercise will help to balance the hormone system in a productive way. Kneel at the back of a chair, with the chair about three feet away from you, so that you can take hold of the upright bars of the back, one in each hand. Hands, as well as body, are to be perfectly relaxed, keeping the spinal column firm. Inhale fully and deeply, at the same time tightening the grasp upon the bars of the chair. Inhale as long as conveniently possible, without the use of effort and without causing unpleasant feelings in any part of the body. Retain the breath as long as you can with ease, still holding tightly to the chair, and, as you exhale gradually, release your hold upon the bars. Exercise in this position for three minutes at a time, but not more than three times per day, although there is no reason why this exercise should not be done during the evening.

During this exercise there is no need to feel alarmed over the peculiar sensation starting at the navel and spreading upwards through the spinal region to the top of the head, as well as downward to the lower extremities of the body. This peculiar warmth is caused by the generation of electric energy in the nervous system, and the cool, fanning sensation felt about the body is the magnetic circle emanating from the innermost soul.

This position will bring tranquillity and calmness. The effect it has on you remains for you to experience. But you must not overdo it, as it is a very powerful exercise. As soon as you begin to feel the chair move, and your knees appear to lose touch with the floor, release the hands at once from the chair and stop the exercise for that day. The curing qualities of this exercise must be experienced and cannot be explained. Things you were unable to comprehend before will begin to appear very simple. In fact, the mind is cleared and you will be able to grasp and understand issues that previously appeared unclear and muddled. Remaining in the position described, with all thought banished from your mind, follow the current of inhalation as it enters the nostrils. For a few moments forget all, breathe evenly and *relax*.

Mentally and physically, exercise is beneficial. Exercise is vital for an all-over sense of well-being. A 20-minute early morning swim, or a brisk walk on a frosty morning, can be very important factors on how you will feel and perform that day. Decide on the kind of exercise you prefer, and which best suits your lifestyle. For older people, of course, the choice may be slightly limited, but even gardening is beneficial. Don't consider it a chore, it is a pleasant way of exercising with the further benefit that it is done in the fresh air.

If you decide to do some of the exercises detailed in my book *Neck and Back Problems*, always keep the following rules in mind: find a comfortable position, keep the spine straight, arms and legs uncrossed and wear loose and comfortable clothes. Always concentrate on the exercise while you are doing it.

A gentle, but nevertheless helpful, exercise is as follows: stretch out in a comfortable position and clench the hands into fists and hold them tightly for half a minute, then relax the body. Tense and relax individual parts of the body in the following order: face, shoulders, back, stomach, pelvis, legs, feet and finally the toes. Hold each part for about half a minute and then relax the body for half a minute. This is a helpful exercise for relieving stress.

Stress can also be relieved by some visualisation techniques.

Withdraw from others and give yourself a little time on your own. Relax and allow the mind to wander. Then visualise yourself as the woman you would like to be. Imagine yourself to be a perfectly healthy and happy woman, and see and believe that you now *are* that woman. You will leave that room in a relaxed and more positive frame of mind.

Categorise exercises that are suitable for the lower body, such as walking, jogging and cycling, and differentiate between these and exercises that involve the upper body, or the whole of the body. For flexibility practise breathing exercises, e.g. tai chi or yoga.

I would also advise some floor exercises, as these can be helpful for strengthening the muscles in the lower back. Where applicable, do the following exercises on a hard surface, covered with a thin mat or a heavy blanket. If it makes you more comfortable, a small pillow may be placed under the neck or in the small of the back. Always remember to start any exercise session slowly to allow the muscles to loosen up gradually.

1. Stand erect while holding on to a table or chair. Bend the knees, straighten up again, relax and repeat the exercise.
2. Lie on your back with your arms above your head and your knees bent. Now move one knee as far as you can towards your chest, and at the same time straighten out the other leg. Go back to the original position with both knees bent and repeat the movements, switching legs. Relax and repeat the exercise.
3. Lie on your back with your arms at your sides and your knees bent. Now bring your knees up to your chest and with your hands clasped, pull your knees towards your chest. Hold for a count of ten, keeping your knees together and your shoulders flat on the mat. Repeat the pulling and holding movement three times. Relax and repeat the exercise.
4. Lie on your back, grasp the right knee with both hands and pull the knee against the chest. Release the knee, then straighten it and relax. Repeat this exercise five times and then do the same thing with the left knee.
5. Bring one knee to the chest, then straighten it, pointing the toes upward as far as possible. Bend the knee back to the chest and return to original position. Alternate the knees with each repetition.

Do only one exercise, ten times per day, during an exercise session first thing in the morning: on the first day do exercise no. 1, on the second day exercise no. 2, etc. After doing the first five exercises for a couple of weeks, start on exercise no. 6, to be followed on successive days by nos 7, 8 and 9. Following the same format then go back from exercise no. 9 to no. 1, again only one exercise per day.

6. With the knees bent, feet flat on the floor and hands clasped behind the head, pinch the buttocks together, pull in the abdomen and flatten the back against the floor. At first, hold this position for a count of five and relax for a further count of five. Gradually increase to a count of twenty. Then do this same exercise with legs extended and arms raised straight overhead.
7. Sit on the floor with the knees bent. Keep the feet flat on the floor, held or hooked under a heavy piece of furniture, to provide leverage. Lie back and cross the arms on your chest, raise both head and shoulders and curl up to a sitting position. Keep the back rounded and pull with the abdominal muscles. Lower yourself slowly.
8. Lie face down, placing your hands on the lower back. Raise the head and shoulders (chest) from a prone position by contracting the back muscles (chin should be raised from the floor as high as possible). Hold this position for a count of five and return to starting position. Repeat this exercise five times.
9. Lie face down and place your hands and arms under the head. Contract the muscles of the lower back and legs by contracting the posterior extensors. Your feet should be raised to 12 inches above the floor. Hold this position for five seconds. Slowly return to starting position and repeat five times.

Hydrotherapy is especially recommended for circulation problems. The following exercise should be done every morning on getting up and each night on retiring. Place a basin of cold water at the side of the bed, and keep a towel handy. When waking in the morning, place both feet in the water. After counting to ten remove the feet from the water and dab them dry. Exercise the toes as if trying to pick up a marble. Do this ten to 30 times. Carry out the same procedure on retiring at night, and you will find that your feet are lovely and warm. It should be understood that this exercise must be done for at least 60 days to feel the full benefit.

Massage, aromatherapy and reflexology are all helpful methods to relieve certain aspects of menopause-induced stress. It must be understood that regular exercise is a vital factor in your life and will give you a new lease of life, never more important than at this stage in a woman's life. It is altogether like turning over a new leaf. The benefits of exercise are that it helps to reduce weight, it diminishes or eliminates muscular aches, pains and stiffness, and leads to an increase in energy levels. Remember that our bodies need physical exercise as much as they require food.

My mother-in-law became very rheumatic during her menopause. Her joints started to swell and she lacked energy badly. This was the more obvious and irksome because she had always been very energetic and industrious. She reacted badly, until she took a grip of the situation and decided on a programme of physical exercise. She made up her mind to go for a swim every morning and also enjoyed a sauna regularly. At home she also took some gentle exercise and before long her rheumatologist quizzed her on what she was doing. To his knowledge she was not taking any medication, although he couldn't fail to notice the changes. His patient now was a much slimmer person, full of energy, and, best of all, without rheumatic complaints.

Much physical tiredness and chronic fatigue is often caused by insufficient physical exercise. While preparing this book, I asked a patient of mine, who just happens to be an extremely fit 91-year-old, how she coped with the menopause. She told me that it was exercise and more exercise that kept her physically and mentally alert and well. She played a little tennis and whenever possible she went for a swim. Now, despite her advanced age, she is still involved in the family business. She is quite a remarkable lady.

This lady's experience demonstrates that many problems can be overcome with determination. It is her belief that regular exercise reduces stress. By keeping busy, she claimed that the menopause symptoms were kept under control. She did, however, mention that during her menopausal years there was little or no talk about menopause-related depression. Nowadays this association is very frequently mentioned. She was intrigued as to why exercise had improved her health and stamina. However, from experience she believed that the secret is found in a combination of diet, exercise and a busy and interesting existence.

You may be able to interest a friend who is willing to join you for a regular swim, ensuring that you encourage each other to stick to the exercise programme.

One of the major worries for women in the menopause is the fear of osteoporosis. Exercise is an effective preventive measure against osteoporosis, as well as against heart and circulatory problems. This is especially the case for women who exercised during the years leading up to the menopause.

In her excellent book *Menopause – the Natural Way*, Dr Sadja Greenwood writes about Giga exercises, designed for contracting and relaxing the muscles that surround the anus, vagina and urethra. This technique was named after a gynaecologist called Giga, and is simple to master, yet very effective. For example, to strengthen the urethra and vaginal muscles squeeze these muscles to the count of three and then relax while passing water. Release the flow of water for three seconds and again squeeze the muscles, alternately squeezing and relaxing a number of times. This may be very simple, but certainly most helpful. Quite a number of these exercises are mentioned in the above book, and they are a worthwhile part of any programme to keep you fit and healthy, at the same time helping to overcome some of the problems of the menopause.

Chapter 13

Relaxation

ONCE, ON A VISIT TO PAKISTAN, an old practitioner taught me something most interesting. He claimed that it is possible to treat all medical conditions from the solar plexus. He substantiated this by telling me that every reflex is concentrated in the solar plexus and can be treated as long as one knows the exact point. Most vital points are concentrated in the solar plexus area around the navel, and certainly this area is very sensitive to relaxation techniques. The vegetative nervous system is centred there and by using the correct technique this can be easily influenced. The exact position of the solar plexus is at the extreme lower end of the sternum or breast bone.

The main branch of the involuntary nervous system leaves the neck at about the third cervical vertebra, travelling down through the entire body and making connections with all the different organs of the interior. Another branch of the nervous system, which is known as the sympathetic trunk, passes down the inside of the body along the spine, connecting the voluntary with the involuntary nervous system, and travels along the ribs and flesh of the body, meeting at the sternum where another connection takes place.

You will see why we have the two terms 'involuntary' and 'sympathetic' for this system. The word 'involuntary' comes from the constant motion of all the organs throughout the body. The word 'sympathetic' refers to the close connection and the working together of so many different plexuses or nerve centres of this system. In the context of the nervous system, the sympathetic and involuntary systems are one and the same, consisting of a group of plexuses or nerve centres which are so interwoven that each is interconnected and supplies energy to the different organs. Each one of the nerves travelling to the different organs is accompanied by a vein which carries the blood to that particular organ.

There are 20 or more of these nerve centres, with nerves extending to the different organs of the body. One plexus supplies the liver, the gall-bladder and the bile ducts with nerve energy and the circulation to these organs is also carried by the vein beside the nerves. Another group carries nerve energy to the heart, the lungs and the bronchial tubes, the nerves branching out from several plexuses to supply energy to the spleen and the pancreas. Again the veins carry the blood to these organs.

Another plexus carries nerve energy to the stomach, the bowels and the duodenum and from this plexus, down a short distance, the nerves come back together again and form two or more plexuses. They extend to the lower part of the back and the lumbar region, forming another nerve centre known as the lumbar ganglion. From here they extend on down into the sacral plexus, the very extreme lower part of the body. These nerves from the sacral plexus travel to the creative organs, fallopian tubes, ovarian glands, uterus, vagina, urinary organs, the bladder and ureter. They extend into the bowels, to the muscles of the anus and the rectal muscles, and pass over the ascending colon to connect with the ileum valve.

The energy automatically leaves the solar plexus, making contact with the different nerve centres, and sending nervous energy to open up congestion in all the different organs. This allows the arteries to force red blood and natural heat up into the body to the various locations that have been out of order. It is quite possible that many of these nerve centres have not functioned properly for some time.

Now, the condition of the nerve centres depends greatly upon the condition of the spine and diaphragm. Remember, if the body is twisted out of shape and if, when running your fingers along the diaphragm, you can feel one rib projecting higher than the other, go to the opposite side and you will find that in the corresponding location, the rib is low and sunken. First the spine must be straight before any permanent relief can be expected. Next, after the spine is straight, the diaphragm, the chest and ribs must be in proper position. If one side of the chest is higher than the other, then you know that there is a part of the nervous system that is under strain and that strain must be released.

It is at this point that I would like to pass on some advice which has stood me in good stead during stressful times in my life. Once, while helping out in a hospital in the Far East, I met a young doctor who was able to perform more operations than any of her colleagues, and yet at the end of the day she still looked fresh. I asked her what her secret was, and she replied that all she did was try to breathe correctly, in order to have an energy supply to draw on whenever needed. She explained that although her method was simple, it still required a bit of understanding.

Where does a new-born baby breathe? You will find that there is little movement in the chest and a rhythmic rise and fall slightly below the navel. As the child grows older and forms its own personality, this breathing pattern will change, usually rising from the naval upwards. Tense people tend to breathe high up in the chest and the same can be said of those suffering from asthma.

The young doctor then told me that her breathing technique was based on 'Hara' and to this day I am grateful that I managed to receive brief instruction in this method of correct breathing. Obviously there are too many exercises to mention here, but I would like to explain the one exercise I practise most days.

About four o'clock in the afternoon, around the time of day I was born, I sometimes begin to feel a little tired. This, by the way, is an experience which many people feel when the time of their birth approaches. I excuse myself for a short while and lie down on the floor and tell myself to relax completely. My eyes are closed and I tell every part of my body, from top to toe, to relax until I feel as if I am sinking deeper and deeper into the floor. Then I place my left hand about half an inch below my navel and place the other hand over it. At that point, a magnetic ring on the vital centre of man – Hara – has been formed. The Chinese have an old saying that the navel is the gate to all happiness and certainly, by doing this, one feels very relaxed. Next I breathe in slowly through the nose, filling my stomach with air and keeping the rib cage still. This sounds easier than it is and actually takes a little time to master properly.

Concentrate the mind on the stomach and breathe in slowly. Once the stomach is filled with air, round the lips and slowly breathe out, pulling the stomach flat. This can be done as often as is desired. Normally, the sensation after finishing this exercise is either one of complete relaxation and a desire for sleep, or of refreshment and a desire to return to work. I must emphasise that the breathing must take place naturally, as a baby breathes. Sometimes it helps to imagine yourself walking in a beautiful garden, where you can smell the wonderful scent of roses which you inhale slowly.

Personally speaking, I always find that this exercise greatly increases my energy flow and I find it of tremendous therapeutic value. It does not require a lot of time, which is another valuable point. I have recommended this method to many patients who were suffering from stress. I have seen it help restore the life force which then helps the body respond.

The Hara breathing technique is very important for relaxing the solar plexus and the vegetative nervous system. Hence, it will relax the whole body as the concentration of energy lies around the navel. It is not as ridiculous as you may think when I advise depressed patients to break into song occasionally, because singing solicits a good vibrationary reaction. Vibration is very important, as is reflected in the phrase 'a simple vibration can shake the entire body into positive action'.

Such positive action requires a clear brain and a well-functioning body, free from aches, pains, constipation and indigestion. In addition: the lymphatic system must be allowed to work unhindered; the skin must be able to carry out its duties without interference; our conscious system must be free from depression; and the liver, gall-bladder, pancreas and spleen must function efficiently. When body, soul and spirit are in harmony, we have positive thoughts. With physical and spiritual vibrations balanced we can translate thought into words. Learning to use words with a raised or elevated vibration will keep us free from dark thoughts. For example, the word 'no' has a heavy vibration. 'No' travels directly to the solar plexus. The word 'yes' is of a higher vibration. The vibration of this word registers in the top of the brain. If you are sitting in a quiet place when you finish your Hara exercises, you can weigh the vibrations and experience that high vibration which will overcome many disagreeable conditions.

Action is like an extremely sensitive conductor, translating and transmitting sounds emanating from the body. The action of the outer and inner eardrum plays a big part in our hearing, and stimulation causes the sense of hearing to be alert. It activates the mastoid gland and is likely to loosen the dead wax in the channel of our ears, clearing the channel and fibrous tissue which conducts the sound. It must be understood that there are several different ways in which our hearing may be impaired. One cause may be the actual hearing organs. On the other hand, it may be lack of judgement or lack of understanding. At times nervousness is responsible for the condition of our hearing. A bad liver or stomach will also cause interference. Impairment may also stem from problems in the cervical region – in other words the bones of our neck may be out of position, causing an impingement or pressure on the nerves leading to the eardrum. In many cases good or bad hearing is controlled by vibration in our environment. There is a big difference between material hearing and spiritual hearing. A major difficulty for the human race is disconnection of body, soul and spirit.

Hearing cannot be confined to the ears. We hear sounds, noises and ringing in our ears, and we also hear the voices of intuition. We all hear the silent voice of temptation, or the voice of our own spiritual consciousness warning us to beware. Some individuals hear things that others never hear. The awakening of a dormant consciousness brings us to a new beginning. The more spiritual light in our hearing organ, the keener and more understandable conditions appear.

Ear problems can cause interference in our hearing, but this, however, can also be lack of concentration. This cause is easily detected. Many people in conversation will ask to have an earlier question or statement repeated. Even if it is not repeated, they will still answer the question. This is merely lack of judgement on the part of the person troubled by hearing. Again people answer with a request to repeat the question. More often than not this is due to a lack of understanding and the cause lies in the thought channel.

Nine-tenths of poor hearing arises from causes not connected with the eardrums or channel in any way, but from influence upon the ears by different vibrations. If a person's thinking is impaired, then his hearing is also impaired. If you cannot think intelligently, then you cannot hear intelligently. There must be perfect union between the five senses, i.e. sight, hearing, touch, taste and smell. These senses are closely related so that when an interference arises in one, it affects the others. Some people may have difficulty with translating what they hear – how often have you heard the expression 'I thought I heard', or 'I thought you said such and such'. Keen thought is interdependent on keen hearing. When a thought strikes the eardrum and is translated properly, we realise what we think with the entire conscious system. We also hear by the vibration of our conscious system – that is why man concentrates on a particular piece of music to be sure that he gets the direct sound, providing proper hearing.

People who appear to be profoundly deaf can prove that as long as life exists in the material body, the hearing is never totally dead. The ears may be in such a condition that sound does not reach the outer or inner eardrum. But there are always two or more locations where hearing can occur, no matter how poor the hearing of the individual appears. By placing a watch against the side of the temporal bone, the individual can hear it ticking, or rather feel the vibration. By taking one end of a solid piece of metal, such as a table knife, between the teeth and resting the other end on a table, the vibration of sound will register distinctly enough on the inner drum for the individual to describe from what source the sound he hears originates – the sound of someone walking across the floor perhaps.

The human body absorbs vibration, just as a sponge absorbs water. If we mingle and associate with people with a low, disagreeable vibration, no matter how careful we are, our conscious system will absorb these vibrations, whether they are positive or negative. Words are stronger than actions. Put in a positive thought, and you will find a positive answer. If you are feeling depressed and miserable, understand that even the smallest positive vibration can alter your situation. Singing, performing or listening to music, or taking note of colours can influence the health pattern of an individual. To this end I hope that we have learned something of the vibratory nature of our make-up and especially about the role performed by our mind and emotions in the menopause.

Exercise and relaxation cause the cells to flush with oxygen. The latter is a transmitter of energy, and, working as a catalyst, it causes the release of energy within the cell. Exercise and relaxation give greater energy release, so that the cell can change from one state to another. These cells should be in harmony with each other or life will cease. Overcoming stress and relaxation will help to ensure a positive effect on the hormone system.

Some of the relaxation methods I have taught have been very successful in helping people to cope with stressful situations. Hot flushes, anxiety attacks and lack of confidence become less destructive as a result of having practised some relaxation techniques. There is no need to choose a complicated programme, because simple breathing exercises can be very effective. After all, breathing is life, because without breathing there is no life. At birth God gave us the ability to breathe and I remind you of an old Chinese saying: 'Deep breathing cleanses the mind and lengthens life.'

You may think that breathing is an automatic action, and, unless something is wrong, we never give a second thought to the actual action of breathing. Remember that babies breathe from deep in their abdomen, which is the correct way (see earlier). How then do we explain that most adults only breathe from the upper part of the body?

A simple exercise is to lie prone and relax the muscles. Concentrate on relaxing the stomach muscles, then breathe in and out by moving the stomach. Continue breathing in and out slowly, concentrating on the stomach. If working on the vibrations, one should use the 'pee-eff-eff' sound as this sound relaxes the stomach muscles.

Patients have found a great improvement in the endocrine system and the hormonal system as a result of these exercises, and during the menopause especially this is a reason to be grateful. The hypothalamus, which is the centre of the endocrine system, greatly benefits from breathing exercises. The art of good breathing is primarily in the exhaling, not in the inhaling. The breath of life is given to all of us, but how we do it is important. People who suffer from hyperventilation must learn to exhale in a controlled manner. Before going to sleep practise rhythmical breathing. For example count to five when you breathe out and take a further count of five before breathing in. Doing this in a controlled manner for a few minutes can ensure a much more relaxed sleep. As is so often the case, simple things can successfully reduce stress and increase overall relaxation. Make a decision to take life a bit easier and if you learn to relax every now and then you will be able to cope better with life and accept it as an ongoing challenge, both physically and psychologically. This challenge is actually a good stimulation, showing that you can do better. If you have achieved the ability to relax by mastering some of these simple exercises, then you know that you can cope with the effects of the menopause.

Never consider yourself to be alone in what you are experiencing, because there are many women going through the same thing. The only difference is that every woman battles or copes with it in her own way. Isolation adds to the stress but with the help of some of these relaxation techniques, many women have managed to get rid of their inner tensions. Always remember that relaxation can help in more ways than one. It is calming and helps to allay fears, while balancing the hormone system and minimising stressful situations that may be encountered.

Actually, planning anything in this line will be of great help. If you notice yourself to be unusually passive, focus the mind on breathing and visualisation exercises and you will soon find the energy to put the mind in gear again. Following some of these tips may encourage you into becoming the woman you would like to be.

Chapter 14

Life Begins at 50 – A New Image

FORTUNATELY, WOMEN NOWADAYS are becoming increasingly conscious of the importance of health and being better informed on the subject helps to allay some of the fears that plagued previous generations. Those generations gritted their teeth and suffered the consequences. It is no wonder that in those days the term 'change of life' indicated the end of something, and held no promise of a new beginning. Nowadays, this time in the life of a woman most definitely indicates a new beginning. Physically, the end of her reproductive years allows her much greater freedom. No longer will she have to check the dates of her monthly cycle when she is planning a weekend away, or a holiday. There is no longer a need to use birth control methods. She no longer experiences the mood swings that are difficult to explain to husband or family, or many of the symptoms that occur during the reproductive cycle. After the menopause women can look forward to a new beginning. Approach this period with a positive outlook and be determined to make the most of it.

I would like to use this final chapter to reiterate briefly some of the advice that can be found in more detail elsewhere in this book. Never think that problems arising from the menopause must be suffered and that, in time, they will sort themselves out. I have mentioned several of the natural remedies which are of great help for specific menopausal symptoms. Also bear in mind that these natural remedies are safe to use because they have no known contraindications.

Also I would like to remind you of the importance of self-examination. Pick any date of the month, it may be the first Sunday in the month or the middle or the end of the month, and examine your breasts. Remember that immediately after a menstrual period the breasts are softest and least lumpy. It is important to do this regularly, and by doing it at the same time every month, you will recognise the characteristics that are peculiar to your breasts. Such self-examination should be done while lying down in bed or in the bath. Fold one arm under the head and with the other hand examine the opposite breast, starting with the nipple and working your way around the breast. This examination should be done with the fingers flat, in small circular movements. Then, lowering the arm along the side of the body, remember to check the area nearest the armpit. When both breasts have been checked stand up and look in the mirror to see if you are aware of any changes in shape, skin, or nipples.

Another very important check is the cervical smear test, which is usually done by your doctor. If this check is not done on a regular basis, please ask your doctor about it. This test is important because there is a good chance of detecting changes in cells before they become cancerous. Some years before cancer of the cervix develops, changes in the cells of the cervix can be detected by microscopic tests. Treatment in the early stages of cervical cancer has a great chance of success.

I have already warned against the pessimistic approach when it is only too easy to blame each and every health irregularity on the menopause. It may be worthwhile, if some of the symptoms cannot be overcome, to try changing some habits in your lifestyle. Headaches, constipation or sleeplessness are not necessarily linked to the menopause, and a reason for such symptoms may well be found elsewhere.

In a recent survey I read that many women in their fifties profess to feeling young and consider themselves fortunate in that they are more able to do as they wish. In most cases their families have grown up and left home, which leaves them with more time for themselves. In these cases it is much easier to decide to go for a daily swim, for example. With a growing family such a decision is much more difficult to carry out. You may prefer to join a yoga class, or go folk dancing. This may be the ideal opportunity to do some voluntary work. In fact, the sooner you realise that the world is your oyster, the better. Reaching the age of 50 gives you the enviable combination of still being young, while at the same time being able to draw on your experience. In a nutshell, you are old enough to know what you would like to do, and still young enough to strive for it. It is the state of mind at this stage in your life that is all important.

The Ladycare 2000 survey report mentioned in earlier chapters contains some contradictory findings. Apparently only eight per cent declared themselves to be concerned about growing old, while 39 per cent did not profess any concern at all. Oddly, the main concerns were expressed by the 18 to 25 age group. Outward signs of impending old age seemed to cause very little concern, and were largely classified as cosmetic inconveniences which would have to be dealt with: only nine per cent worried about turning grey and 19 per cent were concerned at the thought of wrinkles. Most of the worries surrounded the more important issues, such as loss of mental agility (54 per cent) and reduced mobility (48 per cent). Intriguingly, 41 per cent of the younger women acknowledged a concern about loneliness, while the more mature group indicated the onset of ill health as their major concern.

Recently, in the Netherlands, the first private centre for meno-pause-related complaints was opened, creating much interest. The founding gynaecologist says that he is aiming his attention at women who are struggling with hot flushes and other problems and live in fear of osteoporosis. The centre has very quickly made a good name for itself, but I am doubtful if many of the patients sought help elsewhere before attending the clinic. Much of the advice mentioned in this book is within the reach of anyone and can be easily followed. It is my profound belief that women can do more to positively influence their condition by self-help and personal consideration than they can by paying for expensive forms of treatment. The results do not depend on how much is spent, but how it is spent.

Some time ago I spoke to a lady who professed to have been troubled with various symptoms for quite some time, until she read some of the articles in which I mentioned remedies such as Optivite, Dr Vogel's Woman's Formula and Urticalcin. She said that her life had changed since then and she attributed the improvement in her condition to the use of natural remedies.

Yet another lady told me that she did not believe in taking any remedies at all, but she had disciplined herself and no longer drank coffee or alcohol, and she had already stopped smoking some time ago. Together with some dietary changes and some more exercise, she seems to have more or less followed all the recommendations I have discussed in this book. Her menopause came and went virtually unnoticed. That of course is the very best course of action, better still than taking the remedies listed, even though these remedies are free from side-effects. Unfortunately not everyone has the will power necessary to do as this lady did.

The one thing we must firmly believe in is that our health should be as well maintained as possible. This most definitely also applies to the period prior to the menopause, because the healthier one is, the easier it is to cope with the menopause.

Too often a woman's values have centred on the lives of her husband and children. At this stage in a woman's life the children will probably have left home and it is like putting the clock back to the beginning of your marriage. Well, there may be the occasional visit from the grandchildren, but on the whole it is the two of you again, you and your partner. The years around the menopause offer a good opportunity to take stock of the things you have always wanted to do, but have never got around to. Seize this chance and develop an interest of your own, or set aside some time for yourself. In a brochure published by the Scottish Health Education Group I read the following letter:

I started setting aside 30 minutes a day for myself after watching an Australian TV programme. It was trying to persuade people to take time off for themselves and not to feel guilty about it. Well, that message has had the biggest impact on my life. That space in each day just for me helps me keep my sanity and has given me a completely new outlook on life.

Compare this outlook to the lady who came to my clinic, and told me that she could not stop crying because she could only think of her lost youth and that all the good things were now in the past. How sad a predicament for this person because we should look to the future with hope and the desire to make the best of it. The past is over and done with, and now it is time to look forward to what tomorrow may bring. Life still has so many good things in store. Be determined to become the woman you have always wanted to be.

A report from the National Osteoporosis Society stated that teenagers need 700mg of calcium a day, adult women 1000mg, pregnant women 1200mg, and post-menopausal women 1500mg. There are many foods with a good calcium content. For example, spinach contains 600mg of calcium per 100g, and is possibly the richest source of calcium, but all dark green leafy vegetables are rich in calcium. So are kidney beans, dried figs, soya, brazil nuts, lemons, salmon and sardines, for that matter. It is only a measure of common sense that is required, and if you have read any of my other books you may have come across my statement that 'there is nothing common about common sense'.

Please take note of the advice on breathing exercises in order to reduce stress. I have explained the importance of the solar plexus as the centre of the hormone system. It is unhealthy to allow this system to function under a permanent state of tension. For example, the feet and ankles will quickly become swollen. The whole system can be compared to a telephone switchboard. A flashing light indicates an incoming call. Yet, it is not the light that is important, this is only an indicator of action. The circuit is more important, because that allows the call to be connected through.

Remember what I have said about hands being excellent tools for relieving tension, and many of the general ways are also applicable to bring relief for some of the menopause symptoms. The hands are not only tools for expressing conscious thoughts; they are far more important as a means of balancing energy, as long as we know how to use them. The hands speak to the conscious mind by means of the contact that they make with the senses. The language of the hand conveys the healing thoughts of every individual. Even the most simple of vibrations can be transmitted through the hands. You may have noticed that when you sing certain notes, the book or sheet music in the hand will vibrate. The vibrations of the hands are communicated through the tissues where the hands touch them. These tissues vibrate at that rate and in that way energy is balanced and health achieved. Just as the tuning fork responds sympathetically to another of its own pitch, when this vibration is communicated through the tissue, the mind responds to vibrations in the body. The vibrations of a positive mind are a form of energy. All vibration is a movement of something in some direction. This is the reason that hands are so important, because those invisible health vibrations in the tissues can be transformed into health and happiness.

Remember that life begins at 50. Make sure that you believe in your new image and positively accept the challenge by enjoying life to the full.

Bibliography

Campion, Kitty, *A Woman's Herbal*, Century Press, London

Gerson, Miryam, *Menopause, A Well Woman Book*, The Montreal Press, Toronto, Canada

Greenwood, Dr Sadja, *Menopause the Natural Way*, MacDonald and Co., London

Hittleman, Richard, *Natural Foods Book*, Workman Publishing Co., New York, USA

Lark, Dr Susan M., *The Menopause Self Help Book*, Celestial Arts, Berkeley, Ca. USA

de Marco, Dr Carolyn, *Take Charge of Your Body*, The Last Laugh Inc., Winlaw, BC, Canada

Melvile, Arabella, *Natural Hormone Health*, Thorsons Publishing Group, Wellinborough, UK

Mervyn, Leonard, *Woman's Change of Life*, Thorsons Publishing Group, Wellingborough, UK

Reuben, Carolyn and Priestly, Dr Joan, *Essential Supplements for Women*, Thorsons, Hammersmith, London

Shreeve, Dr Caroline, *Overcoming the Menopause Naturally*, Arrow Books, London

Vogel, Dr A., *The Nature Doctor*, A. Vogel Verlag, Taufen, Switzerland

Index

126